A Patient's Guide to
Dialysis and Transplantation
Third Edition

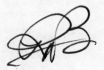

A Patient's Guide to Dialysis and Transplantation

Third Edition

Roger Gabriel
**Renal Physician,
St. Mary's Hospital,
London W2**

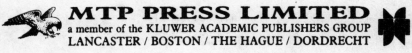
MTP PRESS LIMITED
a member of the KLUWER ACADEMIC PUBLISHERS GROUP
LANCASTER / BOSTON / THE HAGUE / DORDRECHT

Published in the UK and Europe by
MTP Press Limited
Falcon House
Lancaster, England

British Library Cataloguing in Publication Data

Gabriel, Roger
A patient's guide to dialysis and
transplantation.—3rd ed.
1. Renal insufficiency—Treatment.
I. Title
616.6'1406   RC 918.R4

ISBN 0–85200–981–X

Published in the USA by
MTP Press
A division of Kluwer Academic Publishers
101 Philip Drive
Norwell, MA 02061, USA

Library of Congress Cataloguing in Publication Data

Gabriel, Roger.
A patient's guide to dialysis and transplantation.

Includes index.
1. Hemodialysis—Popular works. 2. Kidneys—
Transplantation—Popular works. 3. Renal insufficiency—
Popular works. I. Title. [DNLM: 1. Hemodialysis—
popular works. 2. Kidney—transplantation—popular
works. WJ 378 G118p]
RC901.7.H45G33 1987   617'.461'059   87–3529
ISBN 0–85200–981–X

Printed in Great Britain by
Butler & Tanner Ltd
Frome and London

Contents

CONTENTS

Preface

In many ways this book is a team effort. Many people have helped me in writing it. Firstly, I thank my wife who read the manuscript twice correcting grammatical errors and spelling and clarifying many sentences. Secondly, I thank friends and colleagues at St. Mary's Hospital, including Mrs Jean Emerson, Renal Unit Social Worker and Mrs June Morgan, Senior Dietician, both of whom contributed technical information; Sisters Christine Holmes and Malinie Polpitiye who read and criticized some chapters; Miss Mary Williams, Mr Robert Minor and Mr Richard Viner who as patients read some sections and made useful suggestions. My thanks are due to Miss Veronica Adams who typed most of the manuscript and also to Mrs June Marshall and Miss Joyce Meadows who helped with typing and much photocopying. I must thank Travenol Laboratories Limited whose generous financial support enabled this book to be published. The editorial staff of MTP Press have been very helpful, rapid and efficient in publishing the text.

If any reader wants to know more about renal disease, there

are several good introductory books on renal medicine available. I am sure that the local public library will be pleased to help.

Any parts of this book that are wrong or misleading are my responsibility. If anyone has the energy to point out errors to me I will try to correct them in any subsequent edition.

Preface to third edition

In the five years since the second edition there has been considerable change in renal medicine. Dialysis and transplantation have both improved: hence the need for this edition. The book is meant to be read as a general guide – it should be emphasized that treatment policy varies widely among renal units. In addition, when describing points for or against a particular treatment, I have tried to be neutral or mildly pessimistic so as not to raise false optimism.

Many people have helped in the preparation of this book. As always I thank my wife who has read new portions of manuscript. At St. Mary's Hospital, Sisters Sim Ooi and Lynne Healy have supplied me with technical information on peritoneal dialysis. Mrs Carol Atkins, Senior Dietician and Miss Maureen Miller, Renal Unit Social Worker have helped with their specialised knowledge. Mrs Peggy Peck, a patient, read a new chapter and made useful suggestions. New text has been typed and photocopied by Mrs Wendy Bowers. The illustrator, Mrs Gillian Oliver has supplied six new figures. Travenol Laboratories Ltd.

have generously supported this edition so that it may be freely distributed in Britain. Dr B. A. Bradley of UK transplant and the Registry of EDTA have given permission for me to quote some of their data. Again the editorial staff of MTP Press have been very rapid in production of this book.

June 1987   ROGER GABRIEL
St Mary's Hospital
London W2

1

Introduction

Fifty to eighty people per million of the population develop permanent kidney failure each year. Many of these are between the ages of 15 and 70 years, have families to bring up or other useful parts to play in the community. Without dialysis treatment they would die. During the 1960s and early 1970s centres were set up across the country for their treatment. Most people in Britain know of artificial kidneys and have read in newspapers about kidney transplants. It is vaguely thought that either of these treatments restores a person to normal. Unfortunately this is not necessarily the case and in part this book is written to explain what a kidney patient may need to do and what he can expect. Patients with kidney failure need to know much more about their treatment than someone with arthritis or stomach ulcers.

Dialysis is not an easy way of life. Patients who understand their treatment and are able to co-operate fully tend to be healthier than those who know less about their condition. Dialysis or transplantation requires more from a patient than the treatment of any other medical or surgical disease. The treatment of renal failure affects not only the patient but also his spouse, children, friends and way of life. This book explains some of the problems and suggests ways to help. Success in treatment of permanent kidney failure depends much on the attitude and determination of the patient. This attitude comes in part from knowing what to expect and in this short book is an outline of the treatments available.

When reading this book it should be remembered that different renal nurses and physicians have different policies, use different equipment and often have trained in different centres. Their advice may therefore conflict to some extent with that given here. The local policy will be the one relevant to a particular patient. The number of patients being dialysed in Great Britain is gradually increasing and from 1973 dialysis in America has rapidly increased since Medicare began funding the treatment. This book is applicable to dialysis patients, their families and friends in both countries.

2

Glossary of technical terms

There are many technical terms in renal medicine. A patient has to learn a number of these to obtain an adequate understanding of his treatment. Because many kidney treatments are performed by patients in their own homes a good grasp of technical terms is essential. This chapter defines the terms used in this book. It is intended for reference when reading other chapters. In addition each technical term in the book is defined in the chapter where it is first used. To understand a particular term it may be necessary to look up the meaning of other terms because some definitions rely upon understanding the meanings of others.

acute   In a medical sense this means sudden. For example, a person who had a heart attack develops an acute illness.

'alarm'   An 'alarm' is a high pitched noise made by a kidney machine when a fault has developed. When the fault is corrected the 'alarm' noise stops and dialysis re-starts.

aluminium hydroxide (Aludrox, Alu-Caps) This is a drug required by many dialysis patients to diminish absorption of phosphate from their intestines. A fuller description is given on page 60.

anaemia Anaemia is a deficiency of red blood cells. The majority of people with chronic renal failure are anaemic.

anatomy The study of the structure of the organs of the body.

artery A blood vessel that carries blood away from the heart.

artificial kidney This is a slang term which includes the kidney machine, the connecting tubes ('lines') and the dialyser (see below).

aseptic A surgeon performs operations under aseptic conditions. This means that the gloves, gown and instruments used are sterile, having been specially treated to remove all germs.

bacteria The medical word for germs. Bacteria are found everywhere, including on the skin.

blood group Everybody has one of four main blood groups – O, A, B and AB. Group B blood will cause a severe reaction if transfused into a person with blood group A. In a similar manner the blood groups of persons giving and receiving a kidney are important because they have to be the same. If different, the transplant kidney would be very rapidly rejected.

blood pump The blood pump is used during haemodialysis to pump blood from the patient to the dialyser.

bubble trap Just after the dialyser there is an expanded portion of the blood line which traps any air that may have got into the system. This is shown in Figure 5.8, page 52.

cabin In the context of home dialysis a cabin is a portable room equipped with apparatus for dialysis and placed in a patient's garden.

catheter A catheter is a tube, usually made of silicone.

chronic This is a medical term meaning prolonged, lasting for years. The word also usually implies that the condition will not get better.

chronic dialysis Chronic dialysis is the treatment of chronic renal failure.

chronic renal failure A condition in which the kidneys have been destroyed by disease and can no longer work adequately. This may be shortened to CRF. The term 'end stage renal disease' (abbreviated to ESRD) means the same as very advanced CRF.

Cimino In 1966 Dr James Cimino thought of, and developed, this type of fistula used for dialysis.

continuous ambulatory peritoneal dialysis (CAPD) Dialysis technique carried on continuously while the patient goes about his usual activities. It is described in Chapter 9, page 77.

continuous cycle peritoneal dialysis (CCPD) A form of dialysis used to treat chronic renal failure. A person usually treats himself at home, overnight using a semi-automatic machine whilst asleep. CCPD is described in Chapter 11, page 93.

creatinine Creatinine is a normal waste material produced in the body and removed by the kidneys. A quick and fairly accurate guide to the filtration efficiency of the kidneys is obtained by measuring the amount of creatinine in the blood. A more precise measurement of kidney function can be gained by measuring blood *and* urine creatinine. This is called creatinine clearance.

cyclosporin This is a powerful, expensive, useful drug used in almost all patients to prevent rejection of transplant kidneys.

deionizer Tap water must be purified before it passes into a kidney machine. This removes some calcium salts ('hard' water) and produces 'soft' water. The apparatus which does this is the deionizer.

dialysate; dialysing solution This is a mixture of water and salts which are used for the process of dialysis.

dialysate concentrate This is a concentrated solution of dialysate salts which, when mixed with the correct volume of deionized water, forms the dialysate. A concentrate is less bulky to transport than dialysate solution.

dialysis The process of removing waste products from the blood. The waste products diffuse across a semipermeable membrane into the dialysate.

dialyser The apparatus in which dialysis occurs. There are three types: parallel plate, hollow fibre and coil.

diet Diet is a person's food intake. For kidney patients a special diet is usually recommended to reduce the amount of waste products that accumulate in a person with renal failure. (See Chapter 12.)

dwell time   Period of time during which dialysate is left in the abdomen during peritoneal dialysis. This varies according to the type of dialysis.

fistula   Connection between an artery and a vein, usually in the arm, to allow access to the blood stream for haemodialysis. There is a diagram of a fistula on page 47.

fluids   Any liquid that may be consumed. A fluid is not only tea or a soft drink but also includes soup, broth, stew, ice cream, jelly, custard and any food that has a high water content.

formalin (formaldehyde)   Powerful disinfectant used for dialysers and kidney machines. It is harmful to the skin and eyes so care must be taken when handling it.

glomerulonephritis ('nephritis')   Kidney inflammation, not caused by bacteria, which chiefly affects the filtering parts of the kidneys. Nephritis is a common cause of renal failure.

haemoglobin   The oxygen-carrying part of the blood; contained in the red blood cells.

haemodialysis   The process of removing waste products from the blood using an artificial kidney. There is a diagram of the system on page 52.

heparin   A drug used during haemodialysis to prevent blood clotting in the 'lines' and dialyser.

hepatitis   An inflammation of the liver. In renal units the most important hepatitis is caused by hepatitis B virus. This is infectious and may be caught by staff or other patients. Hepatitis B virus infection is now very rare in British renal units because very careful precautions are taken.

17

heparin pump The pump used to inject heparin into the 'lines' during haemodialysis.

home dialysis The treatment of permanent kidney failure by the patient and spouse in their home using a haemodialysis machine.

hypertension Abnormally high blood pressure.

hypotension Abnormally low blood pressure. A sudden episode of hypotension is not uncommon during haemodialysis.

infection The term used to describe invasion of any part of the body by bacteria, viruses or parasites.

inflammation This is a normal process by which the body deals with an infection or an allergy. If skin is involved it becomes red, warm and painful. Lung infection causes coughing and phlegm without pain. If a severe infection develops an abscess occurs which contains pus.

intermittent peritoneal dialysis (IPD) A form of peritoneal dialysis used to treat chronic renal failure. It is performed in the home with aid of a semi-automatic machine. IPD is described in Chapter 10, page 87.

K The chemical symbol for potassium. In renal units potassium is often referred to as 'K'. See 'potassium'.

'lines' Plastic tubes through which blood flows during haemodialysis.

molecule The smallest chemical part of a substance.

'needling' A slang term commonly used in dialysis units. It is the insertion of a needle or needles into a fistula to obtain blood for haemodialysis.

nephron   The filtering unit of a kidney. It is thought that there are about 1 million nephrons in each kidney.

outflow time   Time taken for dialysate to drain out of the abdomen during peritoneal dialysis.

peritoneum   Thin stretchable semipermeable membrane lining the whole of the abdomen.

peritonitis   When bacteria come into contact with the peritoneum an infection develops. This is peritonitis. Pain occurs and the dialysate fluid become murky-white.

peritoneal dialysis   A simple dialysis system using the peritoneum as the semipermeable membrane. Dialysate is run in and out of the abdomen and waste products are gradually removed.

physiology   The study of how the body and its organs work.

polycystic kidney disease   A fairly common condition which has a strong tendency to run in families. Cysts develop in and on the kidneys which gradually compress and destroy the renal substance over a period of years.

potassium   A chemical element present in all living things. In man the blood concentration of potassium must be kept within certain limits for health. Too much potassium in the blood may be fatal. The kidneys normally regulate blood potassium concentration. A lot of potassium may be taken in food, which diseased kidneys cannot excrete. It is therefore important for dialysis patients to avoid foods high in potassium.

protein   A chemical compound forming an important part of all living cells. It is an essential component of food.

Quinton–Scribner The first really successful external shunt for haemodialysis was developed in Seattle by Quinton and Scribner in 1960.

Redy Portable haemodialysis machine weighing about 65 lb, suitable for taking on holiday.

renal Concerning the kidneys.

renal unit That ward of a hospital in which dialysis takes place.

rejection The process by which the body attempts to destroy tissues which are foreign to it. There is always the possibility that a kidney transplant will be rejected.

run-in time Time taken for peritoneal dialysate to run into the abdomen, usually 4–5 minutes.

saline A mixture of salt and water. In the medical use of the word the quantity of salt is about the same as that in blood.

semi-permeable membrane A thin layer of material, usually synthetic, which has many very small gaps or pores. Through these pores waste products pass out from the blood, but blood cells are too large to escape.

shunt A shunt is a surgically created artificial external connection between an artery and a vein. The connection is made with non-irritant sialstic tubes which are joined together end to end when not being used. There is a diagram of a shunt on page 49.

soft water Water that has been treated to reduce the calcium content.

sterile Free from bacteria. This is not the same as clean.

Tenckhoff   In 1968 Dr H. Tenckhoff developed a catheter which was non-irritating, flexible and designed for chronic peritoneal dialysis. These catheters are widely used.

tissue type   Everybody has a tissue type which is inherited like blood groups. The tissue type is identified before transplantation.

ultra-filtration   The method by which fluid is removed from the body during haemodialysis. The pressure in the blood compartment of the dialyser is adjusted so that it is greater than the dialysate compartment pressure. Some fluid is then forced out of the blood into the dialysate.

ultrafiltrate   Fluid removed from the blood.

under-dialysis   A term covering an imprecise state of health when the patient is less well than expected after some weeks of dialysis and no other medical condition is present to explain the impairment in health.

urea   One of the end products of protein metabolism. Urea is removed from the body by the kidneys and is retained in the blood in chronic renal failure. Blood urea is often measured in renal units.

ureter   The tube from kidney to bladder.

urethra   The tube from the bladder to the exterior.

urinary tract   A general term which includes both kidneys, ureters, bladder, urethra and, in men, the prostate gland.

vascular access   A general term referring to the means of connecting the patient's circulation to the haemodialysis machine. It includes fistulae and shunts. Vascular means having to do with blood vessels.

vein A blood vessel through which blood returns to the heart.

wash back At the end of a haemodialysis treatment it is necessary to return blood from the lines and dialyser to the patient. This is achieved by drawing saline into the system which washes the blood back to the patient. After this has been completed a very small quantity of blood is left in the dialyser. This is the residual blood volume.

'washed out' Some patients find after dialysis that they have less energy and are more tired than usual. These symptoms are described as feeling 'washed out'. They follow a dialysis that has been too 'fierce'. No harm results.

3

Structure and function of normal kidneys

Understanding life with renal failure depends in part upon having a general understanding of how normal kidneys work. This chapter sets out very briefly the structure and function of the waterworks.

A few definitions will help make this chapter clear.

(1) *Urinary tract*. This term includes the kidneys, the ureters or tubes connecting them to the bladder, the bladder and the urethra – the tube which passes to the outside.

(2) *Anatomy*. This means the structure of the body or portions of it such as the urinary tract.

(3) *Physiology*. Physiology is the study of how the body or parts of the body work.

Anatomy of the Urinary Tract

The urinary tract is made up of the kidneys, ureters, bladder and urethra. These are shown in Figure 3.1. The kidneys are at the very back of the body cavity so that their upper portions are behind the lower ribs. Each kidney weighs about a quarter of a pound. Blood flows to the kidneys via the renal arteries and returns to the general circulation through the renal veins. A fine tube, called the ureter, passes down from each kidney to the bladder. Urine passes to the bladder through the ureters. The tube

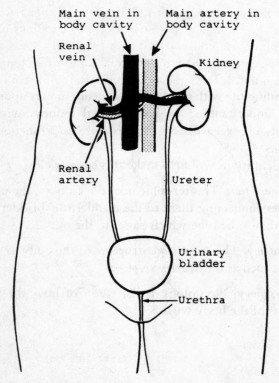

Figure 3.1 A diagram of the urinary tract

through which urine passes out of the body is called the urethra.

The kidney is a very complicated organ. It filters waste products from the blood and forms urine. The filter units of the kidneys are called nephrons. There are thought to be about one million nephrons in each kidney. If too many nephrons are damaged kidney failure develops.

Physiology of the Kidneys

The most obvious function of the kidneys is to make urine. Blood flows through the nephrons which extract waste products and keep necessary substances within the body. The amount of urine made each day is about 1–2 pints. The volume of urine is important and so are the substances it contains. Waste products extracted from the blood are concentrated into the urine. This ability to concentrate substances is vital to normal kidney function. Failing kidneys tend to lose their ability to concentrate and remove waste products.

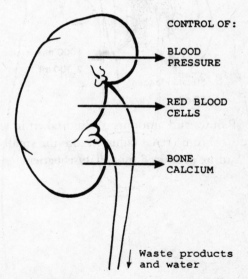

Figure 3.2   A diagrammatic representation of renal physiology

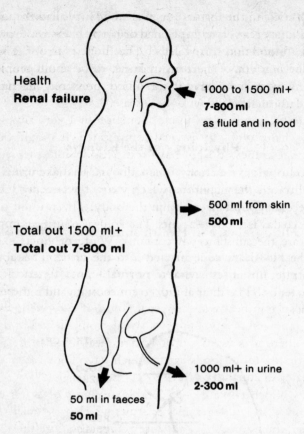

Health
Renal failure

1000 to 1500 ml+
7-800 ml
as fluid and in food

500 ml from skin
500 ml

Total out 1500 ml+
Total out 7-800 ml

1000 ml+ in urine
2-300 ml

50 ml in faeces
50 ml

Figure 3.3 Routes and amounts of fluid taken in and excreted in health and in chronic renal failure. Note the small quantity of urine produced by a dialysis patient

In addition to the formation of urine kidneys have other functions. They are involved in regulating blood pressure. They influence the production of red cells by the bone marrow. They also affect the amount of calcium in bone. As a result people with kidney disease may have high blood pressure, anaemia (not enough red blood cells) or bone disease.

Figure 3.2 summarizes kidney function in a very simple way. In fact renal physiology is very complicated. It should be mentioned that kidneys do not have rest periods but work continuously. This is very different from the artificial kidney which is used only for a very few hours each week (see page 69).

Fluid Balance in Health and in Renal Failure

One important difference between a healthy person and a dialysis patient is the amount of urine passed and the amount of fluid which is safe to take. Figure 3.3 is a diagram showing the differences in fluid balance in health and in renal failure. Everyone loses about 500 ml (approximately 1 pint) as sweat from their skin daily. In hot weather more sweat is produced. In health, the more a person drinks or the more foods eaten which have high water content the greater the quantity of urine.

Foods which contain considerable amounts of water include mince, meat stews, vegetables or fruits which are stewed.

When kidneys reach an advanced stage of failure they lose the ability to produce urine. Drinking water or any other fluid will not 'force' production of urine. Because of this, the amount of fluid that a dialysis patient may safely take, is limited. This is shown in Figure 3.3.

4

Causes and symptoms of kidney failure

Introduction

The term chronic renal failure means persistent reduction in the work done by the kidneys through some disease which cannot be made better by medical treatment. In some cases the disease may leave the patient with some renal function, but for those people who will require treatment by dialysis the damage to their kidneys is progressive until little or no function remains. However, only a small proportion of the population of Great Britain develops sufficiently severe renal disease to need dialysis treatment – about 60–70 adults per million of the population each year and about 2 children in each million each year. Usually the development of renal failure is painless and no symptoms directly related to the kidney disease occur until kidney function falls to 10 per cent of normal or less.

Perhaps surprisingly, the volume of urine passed each day does not change much as the kidney disease advances. However, the quantity of waste products in the urine decreases and these substances increase in concentration in the blood because they are not adequately removed by the kidneys. It is the retention in the body of these waste materials that directly or indirectly causes the symptoms of chronic renal failure.

The rate of deterioration of renal function is very variable, ranging from more than ten years to only a few months. If, as often happens, a person only becomes aware of kidney disease in the late stage of the condition the doctor can only guess as to when it started.

Causes of Chronic Renal Failure

In one sense the cause of a person's kidney failure is not important because dialysis treatment is the same regardless of the reason for the kidney failure. Nevertheless the cause of the renal damage is of interest to the person concerned and may be of importance if a kidney transplant operation is planned.

Glomerulonephritis (often referred to as 'nephritis')

This group of diseases accounts for renal failure in almost half the patients who require dialysis treatment. The disease is caused by persistent inflammation of the nephrons of the kidney. The inflammation leads to damage and scarring so that the nephrons wither away. Proteins from the blood leak into the urine.

The nephrons are the filters of the kidneys and if the inflammation is widespread many nephrons are lost and the kidneys become unable to filter sufficient water and waste products. Symptoms then begin to develop. The inflammation is not due to bacteria but is caused in a very complex manner by the body's immune processes. Nephritis is a painless disease and may exist for years without the person being aware of its presence. Unfortunately it is often not possible to stop the disease process.

Diabetes

This condition affects 1–2 per cent of the population of Great Britain. Apart from raised levels of blood sugar, an important feature of this disease is the damage which occurs to blood vessels. Very small blood vessels are particularly affected – in all parts of the body. Kidneys contain very many small blood vessels and if they are sufficiently damaged renal failure develops. Gradually blood vessels supplying nephrons become blocked and the nephron fades and is replaced with scar tissue.

While there are many people with diabetes only in a very small proportion are the kidneys seriously damaged. Nevertheless a quarter of the people receiving dialysis have diabetic renal failure.

Hypertension

High blood pressure is quite common in Western Europe – at least 10 per cent of adults have some degree of raised blood pressure. However, only very few people with even severely raised blood pressure need dialysis treatment.

In any person with hypertension blood vessels, especially small blood vessels, become damaged. Roughly speaking the higher the pressure and the longer it has been raised, the more blood vessel damage is likely to have occurred. The kidneys contain many miles of very small blood vessels; it is therefore not surprising that sustained high blood pressure may damage the kidneys. In a small proportion of such people the damage is so severe that the small blood vessels of the kidney become irreparable and renal failure develops.

Hypertension which is so severe as to cause renal failure is often called accelerated hypertension. The process is often complex because people with nephritis frequently develop raised blood pressure which may be severe. The kidney damage is then a mixture of that due to the nephritis and that due to the hypertension.

Polycystic Renal Disease

This condition is fairly common. There is a strong tendency for it to run in families: that is, a father or mother may transmit the disease to his or her children. Nearly always both kidneys are affected. Cysts develop in and upon the kidneys (Figure 4.1). Very gradually the cysts enlarge, some to an inch or more in diameter, compressing the normal kidney tissue and slowly reducing renal function. This process takes twenty or more years during which the kidneys may increase fourfold in size.

The majority of people with polycystic kidneys develop terminal, that is, total, renal failure, unlike glomerulonephritis, hypertension and diabetes, in each of which only a few patients will eventually require dialysis.

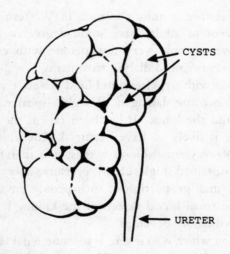

CYSTS

URETER

Figure 4.1 A diagram of a polycystic kidney

Miscellaneous Causes of Renal Failure

There are more than 30 different causes of renal failure and the above outline has only covered the more common. Others are worth mention:

Chronic Pyelonephritis

This condition occurs much more frequently in women than in men. The cause is poorly understood. It is thought to be due to infections of the kidneys in childhood perhaps unnoticed at the time by child or parents. The infection does not always fully die away and may smoulder for fifteen years or more without causing symptoms. With the inflammation scars develop which gradually distort and destroy the kidney substance (see Figure 4.2). The disease spontaneously ceases to progress in the majority of children, teenagers and women, but in a few continued destruction of the kidney leads to chronic renal failure.

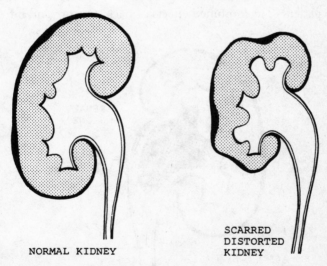

NORMAL KIDNEY

SCARRED
DISTORTED
KIDNEY

Figure 4.2 The normal kidney on the left contrasts with distorted, scarred and shrunken pyelonephritic kidney shown on the right

Obstruction to Urine Flow

If there is persistent partial obstruction to the passage of urine, back pressure develops between the obstruction and the kidney. The kidneys cannot produce urine continually under pressure and will eventually begin to fail. There are three fairly common causes of this kind of renal failure:

Kidney stones

Some people have the misfortune to develop stones in the renal pelvis (Figure 4.3). If small, these may pass out in the urine, but others may become stuck in the ureter (Figure 4.4). If the kidney stone grows larger it will be unable to pass into the ureter but may intermittently block the junction of the renal pelvis with the ureter. Each time an obstruction occurs the kidney is damaged a little bit more.

Kidney stones often develop on both sides. It is perfectly feasible for a surgeon to treat stones but there is a tendency for them to recur. Infection is often present in a kidney affected by stones. In some patients the combined effects of back pressure and infection

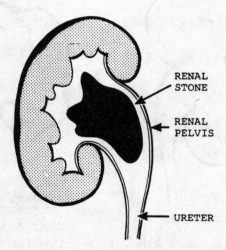

RENAL STONE

RENAL PELVIS

URETER

Figure 4.3 A stone in the renal pelvis

34

cause progressive kidney damage. Some of these patients will require dialysis.

Reflux of urine

This condition is more frequent in children than adults but damage which has begun in childhood may not become evident until adult life. Normally urine in the bladder only goes in one direction – out via the urethra (the tube from the bladder) when the bladder contracts as the person passes urine. In healthy people no urine passes from the bladder back up to the kidneys because the tubes from the kidneys (ureters) are pinched off temporarily by the bladder muscles as they squeeze the urine down the urethra.

In some people the ureters develop abnormally and connect with the bladder in such a way that they cannot be pinched off when the person passes urine (Figure 4.5). In this state urine passes from the bladder in two directions – some down the urethra and

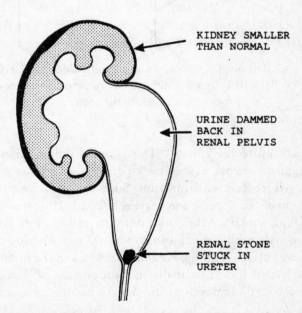

KIDNEY SMALLER
THAN NORMAL

URINE DAMMED
BACK IN
RENAL PELVIS

RENAL STONE
STUCK IN
URETER

Figure 4.4   An obstructed kidney due to a stone lodged in the ureter

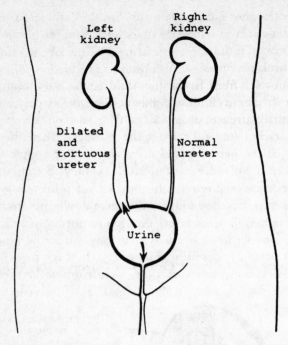

Figure 4.5 The diagram shows a normal right kidney and a damaged left kidney. The left kidney has suffered due to persistent reflux of urine from the bladder up the ureter

some back up to the kidneys. This is called reflux. Kidneys are not designed to work against back pressure and persistent reflux may slowly reduce renal function. Such loss of function is particularly likely to occur if the urine is infected. Unfortunately, in people with urinary reflux, infections are much more common than in people with normal urinary tracts. Over a period of years the ureters enlarge with the continued reflux and the kidneys scar and become smaller. Eventually in a proportion of these people chronic renal failure develops and dialysis becomes necessary.

Urethral valves

A few boys are born with flaps of membrane in the urethra. These cause obstruction to the flow of urine. The urinary stream is poor and the back pressure is transmitted to the bladder, ureters and kidneys. As described in the previous section back pressure and infection are injurious to kidneys. If detected early enough, urethral valves are treatable.

Uncertain Causes

People with chronic renal failure may have no symptoms until their disease is very advanced. Attempts to diagnose the cause of the renal failure in such people may prove impossible.

Frequency of Different Causes of Chronic Renal Failure

Figure 4.6 gives an idea of the frequency of different causes of

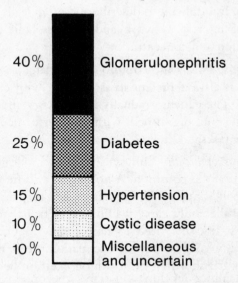

Figure 4.6 The approximate frequency of different causes of chronic renal failure

37

chronic renal failure. Again it should be emphasized that only a very small proportion of people with these diseases will require dialysis treatment. It is of some interest that younger dialysis patients are likely to have nephritis or hypertension.

Symptoms of Chronic Renal Failure

There are no symptoms of chronic renal failure which are caused directly by the kidney disease. It is quite common to meet young patients who have less than 10 per cent of their kidney function left but have no symptoms. In contrast, symptoms are likely to occur earlier in people aged 50–60 years.

The following symptoms may occur in people with chronic renal failure but not all will occur in any one person. In most people symptoms come on so gradually that it is impossible to be sure when the ill health began.

(1) *Vague ill health.* Most people have this symptom to some degree. It is difficult to describe and often leads to a general lack of interest in work and hobbies, and difficulty in relaxation and concentration.

(2) *Tiredness.* This is also common. It is related to the anaemia which is always present in association with chronic renal failure. The patient gradually loses energy and tends to be irritable and dissatisfied with his performance of even routine tasks.

(3) *Shortness of breath.* This symptom is also caused by the anaemia and is common. A housewife will find that carrying a full shopping basket causes her to pant when previously she could carry it home. A person with a manual job will find the need to take more frequent rests and eventually to give up his occupation. As renal function deteriorates shortness of breath on exertion becomes more noticeable.

(4) *Getting up at night to pass urine.* This is a common nuisance

38

and becomes more troublesome as kidney function diminishes below one tenth of normal. Most healthy people do not have to pass urine between, say, 11 p.m. and 7 a.m. This is because normal kidneys have the ability to reduce the quantity of urine produced during the hours of sleep. Damaged kidneys lose this ability and produce urine at an increased rate in an effort to remove some of the persistently raised quantities of waste products in the blood. The extra amount of urine being made continues throughout the night hours and the person is wakened with a full bladder two or three times.

(5) *Sickness*. The last stages of renal failure are often very unpleasant because of the development of a feeling of sickness. Sickness is often followed by vomiting which may lead to a further reduction in kidney function. Sickness may, at first, be avoided by reducing the amount of protein in the diet (see Chapter 12). Eventually it becomes impossible to control sickness except by dialysis.

(6) *Sexual difficulties*. As renal failure advances some people are less sexually active. There are a number of possible reasons. Since most people have insufficient energy for household or job activities they may also have inadequate energy to take part in sex. With less sexual activity there may be less affectionate behaviour shown to the partner which may be more difficult to cope with than the actual reduction in frequency, or duration of intercourse. If for example, a man who has previously been the initiator in sexual behaviour finds that his potency is reduced he may think of himself as a very diminished person and withdraw his affection. A woman who previously enjoyed a normal sex life may be unable to cope adequately with the demands of her healthy partner because of insufficient energy, heavy periods or anxiety regarding treatment and longterm outlook.

CAPD is a very successful treatment of renal failure (page

83) but requires the permanent insertion of a tube into the abdomen through which dialysis is performed. A woman or man with such a catheter (tube) may feel less attractive because of it. This may be sexually inhibiting to either partner because of its presence or position.

Inability to actively take part in sexual matters may easily lead to marital disharmony. It is helpful if a patient with difficulties of this nature is able freely to discuss his or her fears and failures with a member of the renal unit staff together with the sexual partner. In this manner trust can be built up and matters talked about while seeking solutions.

(7) *Psychological difficulties*. From the above discussion it is not surprising that some people who have persistent problems suffer from frustration, anxiety or depression. These tensions may express themselves in aggression or hostility to relatives, or to nursing or medical staff.

(8) *Side effects of drugs*. A person with renal failure may require a number of drugs to treat or control different conditions. Such people are slightly more at risk of an abnormal drug reaction than patients who have normal kidneys. The risks are not great but consequences may be unpleasant, or only very minor. Ideally therefore only doctors who are trained in renal disease should prescribe for patients with renal failure.

(9) *Miscellaneous problems*. Cramps, usually at night, affect some people with advanced renal failure. Legs may swell up when kidney function is very poor and sometimes it is difficult to get rid of such swelling. When a person reaches the dialysis stage of chronic renal failure itching may develop. This may not be easy to control.

Symptoms Which Improve with Dialysis

Dialysis is treatment by a kidney machine or peritoneal dialysis. The symptom which is most rapidly relieved by dialysis is sickness. This goes after a few days and the appetite returns. After a few weeks of dialysis treatment the amount of urine formed often diminishes to about two cupfuls per day (approximately 400 ml, two-thirds of a pint). There is, therefore, no need to pass urine at night. This advantage is exchanged for the restriction in fluid that is allowed. Generally the daily fluid intake has to be about 3–4 cups (600–800 ml).

The symptoms related to anaemia – tiredness and shortness of breath – tend to improve after some months of regular dialysis because the anaemia is likely to improve in part. Cramps usually disappear in the early days of treatment.

5

Principles of dialysis

Introductions and Definitions

Both haemodialysis and peritoneal dialysis depend upon the same very simple principle.

Human kidneys function as filters and the artificial kidney does the same task. To make this section clear a number of definitions are needed:

Dialyser

This is a device by which waste products are removed from the patient's blood. There are two main compartments of any dialyser – the blood compartment and the dialysate compartment. They are separated by a semipermeable membrane. A diagram of a very basic type of dialyser is shown in Figure 5.1. The figure shows that waste products are removed across the semipermeable membrane.

There are more than 100 different types of dialysers available in various countries but they all work on the same principle.

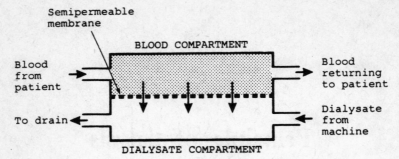

Figure 5.1 A diagram of a dialyser. The arrows represent waste products diffusing, and water ultrafiltrating from blood

Semipermeable Membrane

This membrane is a very thin layer of material which has many minute gaps or pores. Through these pores waste products can pass. The semipermeable membranes are made of cellulose (a product from plants) or from artificial sources. Figure 5.2 is a diagram of a semipermeable membrane magnified many thousand times. Because the pores are of different sizes small substances pass through easily while larger particles pass across slowly or not at all. Blood cells are far too big to cross a semipermeable membrane used in a dialyser. A small substance which easily escapes from blood is urea. The same is true for the salts which are present in blood.

Figures 5.3 and 5.4 show how a semipermeable membrane works. Figure 5.3 shows a glass of water divided into two halves by a semipermeable membrane. Two tablespoons full of cooking salt are put in the left-hand side of the beaker. At first there will be no salt in the right side of the beaker. After a few hours the amount of cooking salt in both halves of the beaker will be equal. This is because the molecules of the salt will diffuse across the semipermeable membrane. It is the diffusion characteristic of the semipermeable membrane which makes haemodialysis possible.

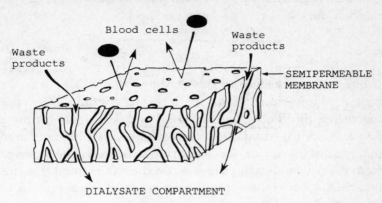

Figure 5.2   A semipermeable membrane magnified many times. It is clear that blood cells are too large to pass across while waste products and water can flow down the pores

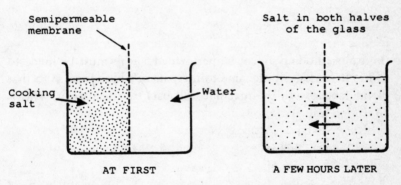

Figure 5.3   The arrows indicate the movement of salt molecules across a semipermeable membrane

Figure 5.4 shows another beaker. The left-hand side is filled with blood taken from a person with chronic renal failure. The right-hand side contains dissolved salts similar to those in normal blood. After a few hours waste products from the patient's blood will diffuse across the semipermeable membrane into the salt solution. The blood will have been partially dialysed. A dialysis machine does the same task but more quickly and conveniently.

Dialysate

Figure 5.1 representing a dialyser shows that half of it is the dialysate compartment. Dialysate is the dialysis fluid. It is water together with dissolved salts identical in concentration to those found in normal blood. Dialysate contains very little potassium (often called 'K' in renal units) so that potassium will be removed from the patient during dialysis across the semipermeable membrane. Dialysate contains no urea or any other waste product so that their removal during dialysis is rapid.

The water used to make dialysate is soft – that is, it contains relatively little calcium. A water softener is used to prepare the water for dialysis fluid.

Vascular Access

Before haemodialysis can be performed a way must be made to connect the dialysis machine to the patient's bloodstream so that blood can flow to the machine and back to the patient. This is

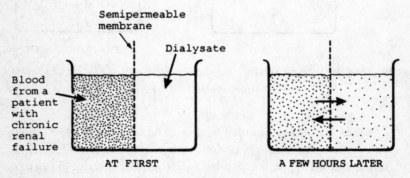

Figure 5.4 Waste products from blood diffusing across a semipermeable membrane

called 'vascular access'. Vascular is an adjective meaning to do with blood vessels. There are two main forms of vascular access:

The fistula

A fistula is a *direct* connection, under the skin, between an artery and a vein. It is made, under local anaesthetic, by sewing a vein in the forearm to the artery that runs down towards the base of the thumb. Some of the blood that previously flowed to the hand then passes directly into the vein (see Figure 5.5). Over the next month the vein grows larger due to the increased quantity of blood passing through it. When the vein has enlarged it is then possible to put wide bore needles through the skin into the fistula to carry blood to and from the dialyser each time the dialysis is

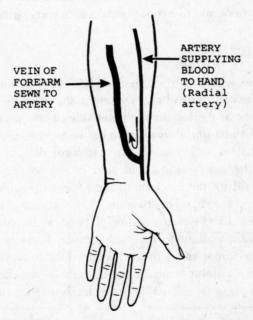

VEIN OF
FOREARM
SEWN TO
ARTERY

ARTERY
SUPPLYING
BLOOD
TO HAND
(Radial
artery)

Figure 5.5 A Cimino fistula. The hand receives an adequate amount of blood because another artery runs down the opposite side of the arm to the radial artery

needed. In a right-handed person the fistula is made in the left forearm and vice versa. This allows the patient to use his 'better' hand to insert needles for himself. Fistulae are used all over the world for vascular access for dialysis.

In some people the veins in the arm are too small to function adequately as a fistula. In this case a length of vein is taken from the thigh and placed under the skin of the arm, one end sewn to the radial artery and the other end to a vein higher up the arm. It is an effective technique.

A fistula can be made in the thigh which functions in the same manner as a forearm fistula. There are certain advantages: both hands are freed for needling; no scars in the arms develop which may be important for women. Also a thigh fistula functions very well for years. Fashioning such fistulae is more complicated. A general anaesthetic and five to seven days in hospital are necessary.

The shunt

For the person who requires urgent dialysis there is not the time to develop a fistula. Instead rapid vascular access can be made by placing a shunt in the leg on the inner side of the ankle (Figure 5.6). A shunt is an *artificial* connection between an artery and vein. It is in two halves which can be separated for dialysis. The end attached to the artery is used to lead blood to the machine. Blood returns from the machine to the patient through the tube connected to the vein. The two ends of the shunt are joined together when dialysis is not taking place. A shunt can be used for dialysis within minutes of its being made. It continues to be used for some time whilst a fistula is created for longer term use. This is because a shunt tends to get in the way of the person's shoes, may separate accidentally and is likely to clot or become infected or both.

Rapid short-term access to the circulation can also be obtained by inserting a special catheter into a large vein which passes behind the collar bone. These are called subclavian catheters. They are

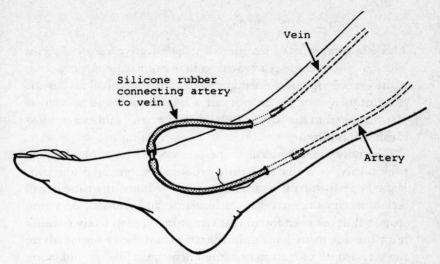

Vein

Silicone rubber
connecting artery
to vein

Artery

Figure 5.6   A shunt inserted into a leg. The shunt is on the outside of
the leg and of the type developed by Quinton and Scribner

inserted under local anaesthetic and may function for two to
three months.

Blood Flow Rate

It is important that a high rate of blood flow is obtained from the
fistula. This is because the efficiency of dialysis is, in part, determined by the quantity of blood that passes through the dialyser.
200 ml per minute is a good flow rate – this is about a cupful of
blood each minute.

Dialysate Flow Rate

A high flow rate of dialysate is also necessary. Generally about
500 ml/minute (nearly one pint) is pumped through the dialyser.

Ultrafiltration

This is a technique which increases the effectiveness of dialysis. The dialysis machine is adjusted so that an increase in pressure is made on one side of the semipermeable membrane. This has the effect of increasing the quantity of waste products and water that is removed from the patient's blood. The extra quantity removed is called ultrafiltrate.

Generally ultrafiltration is performed at the same time as haemodialysis. Water and waste products are removed together. If this is performed too rapidly over a few hours the patient will feel 'washed out', may have a headache and feel sick or vomit (page 73). It has been found that symptoms are less likely to result if a patient is treated with ultrafiltration and then haemodialysis, the total length of treatment being unchanged. This combination is referred to as *sequential ultrafiltration/haemodialysis*. While not necessary for all patients it is of considerable benefit to some.

Needling

Blood has to be taken from the patient to the dialyser and then returned. Blood is taken from the fistula through a wide bore needle (the 'arterial' needle). It is returned through an identical needle to a different part of the fistula (the 'venous' needle). In preparation for dialysis two needles have to be inserted into the fistula. This is shown in Figure 5.7. The positioning of needles in a fistula is often called 'needling' or more correctly cannulation of the fistula. After needling, the needles and the tubes connected to them are secured to the patient's arm with sticky tape.

Single needle dialysis is used in some units. A different type of needle is used which allows blood to flow in two directions at the same time. The principal advantage of this system is that only a single needle has to be inserted.

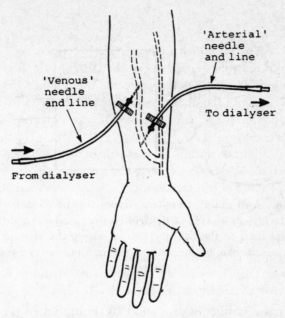

'Arterial'
needle
and line

'Venous'
needle
and line

To dialyser

From dialyser

Figure 5.7   An arm fistula with both needles inserted

Principles of Haemodialysis

There are many different types of kidney machine but all have essential features in common. An outline of the pathways through which blood and dialysate flow is shown in Figure 5.8. The tubes through which the blood passes are called 'lines'. Blood flows from the arm to the dialyser by the arterial line and from the dialyser back to the arm via the venous line. A pump (the blood pump) is nearly always needed to obtain a sufficiently high blood flow rate. Just after the dialyser is an expanded portion of the venous line called the bubble trap. This is a safety device to collect any air that may leak into the circuit.

Dialysate comes from the machine and passes through the dialyser in an opposite direction to that of the blood. The kidney

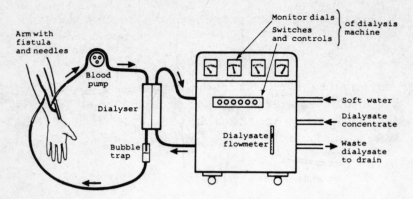

Figure 5.8 A diagram of the basic flow paths of a kidney machine. The blood pathway leads from the arm via the blood pump through the dialyser and back to the fistula. The dialysate pathway extends from the source of dialysate in the machine through the dialyser and then to the drains

machine has a number of dials and looks complicated. These dials are safety devices which continually check different parts of the system. If a fault develops the machine 'alarms'. This means that the machine temporarily switches off, sounds a buzzer and shows a coloured light on the control panel. It is not possible to re-start dialysis until the fault has been corrected. The first sight of a kidney machine with its dials and push-buttons is often daunting. After a few weeks' experience many dialysis patients have learned to sort out the essentials of the system.

Principles of Peritoneal Dialysis

Peritoneal dialysis looks very different from haemodialysis but the basic principle by which it works is the same. Haemodialysis depends upon water and waste products crossing a synthetic semi-permeable membrane. Peritoneal dialysis depends upon water and waste products crossing a naturally occurring semipermeable membrane – the peritoneum.

Here are some definitions to help make this section clear:

Abdominal Cavity

This is in the belly. It contains the liver, stomach and intestines. The kidneys and large blood vessels lie behind this cavity and in front of the spine. Apart from the normal contents there is the space in an adult male to hold about 4–5 litres of fluid.

Peritoneum

The whole of the body cavity is lined by the peritoneum. This is a thin and stretchable membrane which moves with the stomach and intestines. The peritoneum has a large supply of blood which passes through it in very small blood vessels. Normally a little fluid escapes from these blood vessels to lubricate the peritoneum. Peritoneal dialysis is possible because fluid and waste products can cross from the bloodstream through the peritoneum, which

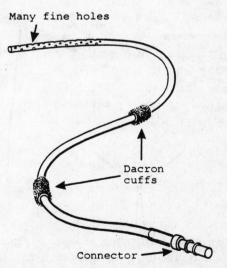

Figure 5.9   A diagram of a chronic peritoneal dialysis catheter

functions as a semipermeable membrane, into dialysate which has been placed in the abdominal cavity.

Catheter

This is a tube with many small holes in its side at one end as shown in Figure 5.9. The catheter is inserted into the belly through a small cut just under the navel. The catheters used for peritoneal dialysis are flexible and non-irritating. They can be used again and again for months or years. They are called Tenckhoff catheters after the doctor who developed them. Figure 5.10 shows such a catheter inserted into the abdominal cavity. Either one or two Dacron cuffs are placed around the catheter when it is manu–

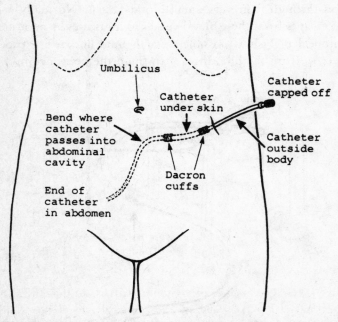

Figure 5.10 A chronic peritoneal dialysis catheter in place. Approximately two thirds of the catheter is under the skin or in the patient's abdomen

factured. They function by causing a painless irritation which leads to development of scar tissue. This tissue helps anchor the catheter to the patient's tissues. For the first month the catheter should be handled with care until it is fully secured by scar tissue.

Dialysate

The dialysate used in peritoneal dialysis is similar to that used for haemodialysis except that it contains a sugar (not the kind used in tea or coffee). The sugar–dialysate solution exerts a 'sucking' effect on the peritoneum which draws out fluid from the patient. The greater the quantity of sugar present the stronger the 'suck' produced.

Peritoneal dialysis is simpler than haemodialysis but takes more

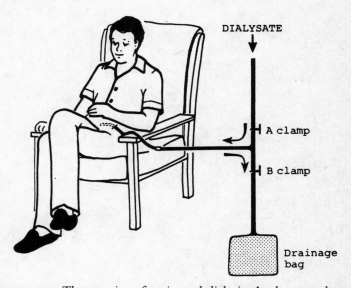

Figure 5.11   The practice of peritoneal dialysis. At the start clamp B is shut and clamp A is opened allowing dialysate to flow into the abdomen. Clamp A is then closed and clamp B opened so that dialysate can flow out of the abdomen. The procedure is then repeated either by hand or machine for a number of hours

time. Dialysis fluid comes either from a semi-automatic peritoneal dialysis machine or in plastic bags containing 1 or 2 litres (about 2 to 4 pints) or larger. Warmed fluid flows down a sterile plastic tube connected to the Tenckhoff catheter into the abdominal cavity. It is left in the abdomen for a period of time to allow transfer of waste products to take place and then it is allowed to run out. The process is repeated many times. The system is shown in Figure 5.11. When a Tenckhoff catheter is first put into a patient it must be used continuously for the first 48 hours. This is to prevent it from becoming blocked. After 48 hours use the catheter can be capped off until the next time it is used.

The precise constitution of dialysate used for peritoneal dialysis can be read from the bags in which the fluid is supplied.

6

Preparation for dialysis

Introduction

This chapter gives an idea of what happens before a patient begins dialysis. It also suggests a few things that are worth thinking about before dialysis treatment starts.

Some people have a few months or years warning that their kidneys are failing. Thus they will have time to get used to the prospect of dialysis and gain some idea of the restriction that it will place on their life. However advanced chronic renal failure may creep on unknown, so that dialysis may be necessary shortly after the diagnosis is made. For people in this group the sudden change in the way of life may be a major shock. Over a period of a few weeks a person has to change from independent life to one of frequent visits to hospital and treatment by a dialysis machine. Even for patients who have had warning this period may prove to be a worrying and stressful time.

Technical Procedures needed before Haemodialysis can be Started

In order to perform haemodialysis a way must be made to connect the dialysis machine to the patient's bloodstream so that blood can flow to the machine and back to the patient. This is called obtaining 'vascular access'. The word vascular is a word meaning to do with blood vessels.

If time allows, a fistula is made when the patient's kidney function has fallen to about one tenth of normal. Fistulae and shunts have been described in the previous chapter on pages 46 to 49. A fistula is an internal connection between an artery and vein in the forearm from which blood can be obtained for dialysis. A shunt is made outside the ankle when there is insufficient time for the creation of a fistula. The shunt can be used immediately after it has been made whereas four or more weeks have to pass before a fistula should be used.

Chronic Peritoneal Dialysis

If peritoneal dialysis is planned, a catheter is inserted into the abdomen. The catheter is a tube made of flexible non-irritant material, of the type developed by Dr Tenckhoff. Dialysate (dialysis fluid) is run into and out of the abdomen through the catheter during the period of dialysis. When a Tenckhoff catheter is inserted it is used immediately and continuously for a period of 48 hours. In this way the chance of the catheter becoming blocked is much reduced. After this it may be used intermittently. There are three main forms of chronic peritoneal dialysis. They are discussed in Chapters 9, 10 and 11.

Diet

At some stage during the gradual loss of kidney function patients will be advised to change some of the foods they eat. Diet in this sense is nothing to do with dieting to lose weight. A diet for a renal patient is to help him avoid some of the symptoms of chronic renal failure (see page 39). The most common and troublesome symptoms controlled in this way are nausea and vomiting.

The main change required is reduction in the protein content of the diet. Many of us eat more meat or fish than is actually necessary for a healthy life. It is therefore possible to reduce protein intake without leading to undernourishment.

After digestion protein is broken down to a substance called urea and other by-products. Urea is normally excreted by the kidneys. In kidney failure the amount of urea in the blood increases and the quantity in the urine decreases. It is not urea itself but other related substances which cause the nausea and vomiting in advanced renal failure. When the dietary protein is reduced the amount of urea and other waste products in the body falls and the person feels better. This is shown in Figure 6.1.

It has only recently been realized that reduction in the amount of urea in the person's blood is directly beneficial. When kidneys gradually fail the number of nephrons (page 30) is reduced and each single nephron has to work 'harder' to excrete urea into

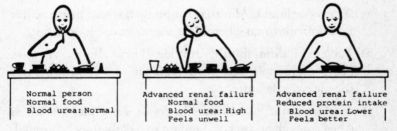

Normal person Normal food Blood urea: Normal	Advanced renal failure Normal food Blood urea: High Feels unwell	Advanced renal failure Reduced protein intake Blood urea: Lower Feels better

Figure 6.1 The improvement in health that may occur in a patient with chronic renal failure when the protein content of the diet is reduced

urine. It is now known that this extra work may increase the rate at which nephrons become scarred and functionless. Therefore if the amount of protein eaten is reduced, less urea is produced and each individual nephron is likely to survive an extra number of months. It is for these reasons – obtaining longer kidney life and setting the time when dialysis will be needed back – that a diet containing a reduced protein content is recommended. This topic is further discussed on page 98.

Drugs

Dialysis patients do not require many drugs when they are well and dialysis is progressing satisfactorily. Almost all substances in the blood are controlled by dialysis so that concentrations do not become too high. The major exception is phosphate. Phosphate is one of the constituents of all foods. It is rapidly excreted by normal kidneys. In kidney failure, phosphate, like urea, builds up in the blood. If there is a persistent high blood concentration of phosphate it can combine with calcium in the blood. The calcium–phosphate mixture is then deposited in blood vessel walls and damages them. Such damage can be avoided if the blood phosphate is kept about normal. There are two drugs which can be taken to reduce the amount of phosphate which is absorbed from the intestines. One is aluminium hydroxide and the other calcium carbonate. Neither is particularly pleasant to take regularly. Aluminium hydroxide comes in three different forms:

(1) As a white liquid (Aludrox; Amphogel) which many people find difficult to take because it leaves an unpleasant taste.

(2) Tablets of aluminium hydroxide. These also are effective but some people find them difficult to swallow because they leave a dry mouth.

(3) As aluminium hydroxide powder in a capsule, known as Alu-Caps. These are large and up to 6 daily may be needed.

Aluminium hydroxide is not prescribed for long periods of

time because a very small quantity of the aluminium is absorbed and deposited in different tissues, notably bone. Small amounts of bone aluminium are unimportant but if a substantial quantity is deposited in bones over a period of years they become weaker. Bone and joint aches develop and fractures may occur. For these reasons aluminium hydroxide is infrequently prescribed for more than one year continuously and the amount of aluminium in the blood is measured regularly. If by mischance too much bone aluminium developed it can be removed by a course of a drug called desferrioxamine for some months.

Calcium carbonate comes in two forms:

(1) As a suspension in water. This is not a satisfactory form of the drug because it does not keep for more than one week.

(2) As tablets. These are the usual form in which this drug is given but the tablets are very dry and up to ten daily may be required.

In most dialysis units calcium carbonate is being used more frequently than a few years ago. Often patients take calcium carbonate or aluminium hydroxide on an alternating basis.

Treatment with one of the preparations of aluminium hydroxide or calcium carbonate is usually begun at the same time as the fistula is created.

Vitamin Tablets

Vitamin tablets are often prescribed for patients either before they begin dialysis or when dialysis treatment has been started. It is not essential to take these every day without fail. In some circumstances vitamin D is necessary. The vitamin is given in the form called One-alpha or Rocaltrol. It is essential that these drugs are taken as prescribed. Vitamin D and calcium carbonate should only be taken together under direct medical supervision.

61

Iron and Folic Acid Tablets

These drugs are also frequently prescribed. The need for them varies from person to person.

Resonium

Resonium, like aluminium hydroxide, is not taken into the body by the intestine. It functions in the large bowel by absorbing potassium (page 19). The potassium, combined with the resonium, is passed out of the body in the motions. Resonium is prescribed when there is a danger of the blood potassium rising too high, for whatever reason (page 100). This drug is a dry sand-like powder and very unpalatable. It is best taken mixed with honey or jam. Although unpleasant to take, Resonium is very effective and maybe life saving.

Holidays

Regular dialysis treatment has to be performed two or three times each week. The longest safe period between dialyses is five days. This long gap should only be taken after medical consultation, with care and not often.

From the above it is obvious that life on dialysis restricts the freedom of the patient. The restriction applies equally to home or hospital, haemodialysis or IPD (page 89), but to a lesser extent to a patient receiving CAPD (page 77) or CCPD (page 93). If a potential dialysis patient has plans for a holiday abroad it should be taken before dialysis treatment begins, if his condition permits. Holiday plans should be talked over with the renal physician because there may be special features of the person's condition which could be important. When on dialysis, weekend holidays are possible. Many renal units have a holiday chalet where the patient may go and stay with family and spouse. These chalets have an artificial kidney in a separate room where the patient can treat himself during the course of his holiday.

Since the mid to late 1970s much progress has been made enabling dialysis patients to take holidays. A CAPD patient can now obtain dialysate in any part of the developed world. Arrangements are made by courtesy of the manufacturer. There are several portable kidney machines so that haemodialysis is possible almost anywhere provided that there is water and electricity. There are also schemes whereby a patient may receive dialysis in a hospital different from his own. Such facilities vary from one country to another.

Other Topics to Consider before Beginning Dialysis

When the diagnosis of renal failure is made the renal physician will explain the plan of treatment to the patient. Most people are at first unable to take in all that is involved in dialysis and possible transplantation. It is a big topic and there are technical points to be understood. In part this book has been written to help patients to go over what their doctors have told them.

In the weeks or months before dialysis the patient should discuss his or her future with various people.

(1) A talk with the patient's spouse and children is important. Some people have a tendency to try to avoid the inevitable by ignoring it. It is better to discuss matters as fully as possible because it is not simply one member of the family who is to be treated. Each member of the family is affected by dialysis and all should have an idea of what will happen. The family will already have felt some effect when the patient became ill; they will suffer fear and anxiety when the diagnosis is made – usually when the family member is absent in hospital. After dialysis begins he or she will then need to attend twice, or thrice weekly for a period of six to eight hours on each occasion. This time together with time spent travelling to and from the renal unit may take up almost two days each week. A lot of leisure time is thus lost. Additionally if home dialysis is planned then a room

will have to be put aside and plumbing installed. All these matters affect the whole family and should be discussed.

(2) The patient's employer will have to be told. Generally employers are very sympathetic to employees who develop chronic renal failure. It may be possible to change the job or the working hours to fit in with dialysis times. If the patient has a heavy job it is best that a lighter job be found. A self-employed person will have to plan how to keep going on a three- or four-day week.

Unfortunately many people on dialysis lose some income because they cannot work full-time. Patients on home dialysis are better able to fit in their dialysis periods with their jobs, housework, shopping and hobbies. CAPD patients enjoy, in some respects, fewer restrictions.

(3) A chat with someone who is already on dialysis treatment may be very useful. Ideas and suggestions from a person who is coping with the difficulties of dialysis will help the new dialysis patient plan his new type of life.

(4) It is a good idea to look for hobbies that can be enjoyed whilst dialysis is being performed. These include reading, writing, listening to the radio, watching television, knitting, sewing, painting – indeed, any hobby that can be enjoyed without requiring much movement.

(5) It is a good idea to join the local branch of the Kidney Patients' Association. By doing so a new patient will meet a number of people who have all learnt how to cope with dialysis, its restrictions and advantages.

(6) No restrictions are placed upon a driver simply because he is a dialysis patient. It is prudent to inform the Insurance Company. Apart from constraints on time made by dialysis a patient can use and enjoy his car like any other driver.

7

Haemodialysis

Introduction

Haemodialysis is one of the most widely used treatments for patients with kidney failure. It is performed at home or in hospital. The part of the hospital which is used for dialysis may be called the renal unit, the dialysis unit, the artificial kidney unit or the haemodialysis unit. Generally a renal unit has about ten beds – often called dialysis stations. In some units and homes patients dialyse sitting in a chair. Usually a hospital dialysis station is used by at least two patients in any 24 hours.

The first sight of a dialysis unit may be frightening because everything appears complicated. Starting dialysis is in some ways like beginning a new job with new people to meet and new routines to learn. Also many people are unwell before their first dialysis and any problem seems greater when one is not fit. After a few weeks the renal unit loses its strangeness and the new patient begins to learn how to dialyse himself.

Renal units are run by nurses. The head nurse will be a senior sister (or, if a man, a charge nurse). She is responsible for organizing the unit as well as nursing the patients. She will be helped by additional sisters, staff nurses and other nursing staff. Large renal units have one or more additional sisters whose job is to visit home dialysis patients (see Chapter 14) and advise CAPD patients.

Renal units are friendly places – most people are on first name terms. Staff try to make the renal unit as pleasant as possible to help patients cope with their problems. It is well understood that haemodialysis affects the patient's whole family, friends and lifestyle.

Technique of Dialysis

The technique of dialysis varies in detail from unit to unit. In this section an outline of the procedure is given. Details have to be learnt in each unit.

Four new definitions are needed. It may also be necessary to look at the previous chapter or the glossary (page 13) for the meaning of other technical terms.

Saline

This is a mixture of water and salt. 'Normal' saline contains salt in about the same amounts as is found in human blood. Saline is delivered to hospitals in sterile plastic containers. The container is labelled showing the contents.

Sterile

This term means the complete absence of bacteria (germs). Sterile is therefore *not* the same as 'clean'. Clean is the absence of dirt; sterile is the absence of bacteria.

Clamps

Haemodialysis is very much concerned with blood and saline flowing through tubes ('lines'). At times it is necessary to interrupt the flow. So that blood or saline will not drip out of a disconnected line it is pinched off by putting a clamp across the line.

Heparin

Blood outside the body will clot. Clotted blood will not flow and cannot be returned to the patient. Heparin is a liquid drug which stops blood from clotting. The effect wears off quite quickly so it has to be used continuously during haemodialysis.

The rest of this chapter covers the main points of haemodialysis technique.

(1) Before the patient arrives the machine will have been self-sterilized. It is then rinsed through with fresh softened water.

(2) The next step is to clip the artificial kidney (dialyser) to a stand and to connect the lines carrying dialysate to and from the machine to the dialyser. Dialysate is then allowed to flow through the dialyser.

(3) Next the blood lines need to be unwrapped from their packets (a fresh sterile set is used at each dialysis) and connected to the 'arterial' and 'venous' ports (entrances) of the dialyser.

(4) A 1 litre plastic bag of salt solution (normal saline) is then attached to the arterial line and the blood pump switched on. The sterile saline solution passes down the arterial line, through the blood compartment of the dialyser and via the venous line to a bucket. When the plastic bag is almost empty the blood pump is switched off. Clamps are placed at each end of the lines. By filling the lines with fluid air is removed and the lines are ready for use.

(5) Whilst the above procedures are done the patient weighs himself and makes a note of the weight. This is the pre-dialysis or 'wet' or 'coming on' weight. The patient also measures and records his blood pressure lying down and standing up.

(6) A sterile tray is prepared containing items that will be required for 'needling'. These are gauze swabs and a few small dishes in which are placed a skin antiseptic solution and a dilute solution of heparin. This is called heparin–saline. A few syringes and needles are placed on the tray together with the 'arterial' and 'venous' needles (see page 50). Local anaesthetic is sucked into one syringe and two others are filled with heparin–saline solution. A fourth is filled with pure heparin – this is the 'loading dose' which is to be given just before dialysis begins. Somewhere close by a few clamps are placed.

(7) A large syringe of heparin is prepared. This is connected by a fine tube to the arterial line. During haemodialysis an infusion pump slowly delivers the heparin into the line to prevent clotting.

(8) The 'arterial' and 'venous' needles have to be inserted into the fistula at about this stage. This is the worst part of dialysis for most patients and causes most anxiety. The forearm is thoroughly cleansed with antiseptic. A small quantity of local anaesthetic is injected under the skin just over the fistula. Next, the fistula needle is pushed through the anaesthetized area into the vein of the fistula. When it is in the correct position a little heparin–saline is injected to keep the needle free of any blood clot, the line from the needle is clamped and the needle and line are secured to the skin with sticky tape. The whole process is then repeated for the second needle. It does not matter whether the 'arterial' or 'venous' needle is inserted first. During the initial weeks of dialysis the patient is 'needled' for each

dialysis by one of the nurses but at the same time the patient is taught how to do it himself. Eventually it is possible for a person to 'needle' himself with only minor aid from a helper. In some units single needles are used which allow blood to flow in opposite directions at the same time.

(9) When the needles or needle are in place the line from the 'arterial' needle is connected to the line to the blood compartment of the dialyser. The clamps are removed, the blood pump switched on at a slow speed and blood will flow from the patient to the artificial kidney. As it does so, it washes out the normal saline in the lines which is caught in a bucket. Around this time the patient injects the loading dose of heparin into himself via the 'venous' needle or the venous part of the single needle.

When the blood passes through the dialyser the saline in the venous line becomes a very faint pink. At this stage the blood pump is switched off. The line from the dialyser is connected to the 'venous' needle and the blood pump switched on. If all is well the heparin pump is then switched on. Dialysis has begun and a note of the time is made.

(10) The blood pressure should be measured and recorded at the beginning of dialysis and at 2-hourly intervals thereafter.

(11) Once a person has started there is a period of 3 to 6 hours during which he is restricted in what he can do. It is a time for reading, listening to the radio, watching television, eating, chatting or playing cards with fellow patients or sleeping.

(12) About 45 minutes before the end of dialysis the heparin pump is switched off.

(13) The procedures at the end of dialysis are approximately the reverse of those when starting.

The blood pump is switched off temporarily. The 'arterial' needle line is clamped and then disconnected from the line to the dialyser. A new bag of saline is attached to the dialyser line. The blood pump is switched on again. Saline is drawn into the system and the blood in the venous line within a few minutes becomes diluted with the saline. This is the 'wash-back' stage. When most of the blood from the dialyser has been washed back into the patient the pump is stopped again and the line from the dialyser to the 'venous' needle is clamped and disconnected. In this way most of the blood is returned to the patient's body.

(14) The patient then, with help, removes both needles from his arm and places dressings over the puncture sites. After a rest the final procedures are to remove the dialyser from its stand, wash and sterilize it, throw away the lines, wash down the machine and set it to self-sterilize.

(15) The patient then takes his lying and standing blood pressures and weighs himself again. This weight is the post-dialysis or 'dry' weight, and is a measure of the success of dialysis in terms of removing fluid (ultrafiltration).

The above is a simplified description of the technique of haemodialysis. Details will vary from unit to unit but are similar whatever machine and dialyser are used, at home or in hospital.

8

Difficulties with Haemodialysis

Everyone involved with dialysis patients knows that the treatment can be very stressful, for some more than others. Many patients have difficulty in adapting to their new way of life. There are the often unspoken fears regarding earning capacity, length of artificially prolonged life and the uncertainties of waiting for a transplant kidney.

Problems associated with haemodialysis can be divided into two groups – technical and psychological. Often these overlap and one can worsen the other. Similar problems trouble people being treated with chronic peritoneal dialysis (see Chapters 9, 10 and 11). In this chapter only the most common difficulties will be discussed.

Technical Problems

Vascular Access

This is the system by which blood is taken from a patient to the machine and then returned. Fistulae and shunts have been described on pages 47 and 48.

In some patients it may take weeks, even with the aid of first-class surgeons, to create an adequate fistula. Some fistulae clot within hours of being made or may clot at a later time. In others the vein does not enlarge sufficiently to use for dialysis. Shunts clot easily. In these circumstances repeated operations are needed. While these operations are minor in themselves repeated failures are depressing and worrying for the patient.

Given time adequate vascular access can always be achieved. During the period of trying to make a good fistula it will not be possible to dialyse adequately and the health of the patient may suffer. This in turn may worsen his anxiety.

Needling

The insertion of needles into a fistula has been described on page 68.

Some fistulae can be very difficult to 'needle' – even by expert nurses. Repeated attempts are therefore needed. This is unpleasant because it is painful, the arm is likely to be bruised and the patient fears that dialysis may prove impossible. Needling tends to become easier in time but, if not, a new fistula has to be made.

Under-dialysis

This is a term used to describe the condition of a patient who is insufficiently well after weeks of technically adequate dialysis during which there has not been the expected improvement in wellbeing. There may be some simple explanation such as an extra anaemia. Often under-dialysis is caused by too few hours of dialysis. The treatment is therefore to increase the length of dialysis and perhaps to dialyse more frequently each week. Under-dialysis is probably caused by insufficient removal of waste products. It may take weeks of extra dialysis to restore the patient's health. Sometimes it is found that the use of a different make of dialyser will aid in improving a person's health.

Hypotension

This term means low blood pressure. If a haemodialysis machine is set so that it removes too much fluid during a dialysis period, the patient's blood pressure will fall below normal. The symptoms are unpleasant and include faintness, nausea and vomiting. It may be possible to avoid hypotension by careful adjustment of the machine. If the patient has poor venous access the pressure in the blood line from the dialyser becomes too high, too much fluid is removed by the artificial kidney and the blood pressure falls. This is easily treated by running in normal saline (see page 66). There are no permanent effects.

Washed out

Quite often patients find that they feel well before haemodialysis but on the day after dialysis they feel more easily tired, have less energy and less interest in life. It is often described as being 'washed out'. This interferes with day-to-day life because they are less well than usual two days each week – assuming that they are dialysed twice weekly. This unpleasant complication is due to the kidney machine being too 'fierce'. During the 4 to 6 hours of dialysis a lot of waste products are removed together with water. The rate of removal is rapid and the person is 'drained'. It takes about a day to recover. Whilst being 'washed out' after dialysis is in one sense a measure of efficient dialysis, having to work in that condition next day is not pleasant. Unfortunately it may not be possible to avoid such symptoms if a person is dialysed twice weekly. It is less likely to occur if the patient has three haemo-dialyses each week.

Infections

Dialysis patients are probably not more likely to catch an infection than anyone else. However, some patients, either due to poor technique whilst 'needling' or due to picking at their fistulae, poke skin bacteria into the bloodstream. This causes an unpleasant illness needing admission to hospital.

Psychological Problems

These are important but can be overcome, particularly if a patient has some idea of what to expect. Dialysis is a way of life affecting a person's job, family life and recreation. The new dialysis patient has first to accept that he has chronic renal failure to such a degree that he can no longer live without an artificial kidney. He may then think that his dialysis will occupy 2 or 3 periods per week, leaving the rest of his life unaffected to proceed normally as before. This is not so. There are three stages in the life of a dialysis patient.

The 'Honeymoon'

Initially there is the interest of learning the technique, when everything is new. The worst symptoms of renal failure (see page 41) rapidly improve so the person feels more cheerful and confident.

Realization of Restrictions

After a while the newness wears off. The patient realizes that he is living but not in full health, has to keep to a limited intake of fluid, must attend hospital twice weekly, cannot go away for normal holidays and may lose some income if he is unable to work full-time or, in the case of a mother, pay someone to help with the children. In addition there may be symptoms such as itching, muscle cramps, poor sleep, or severe thirst.

Some people appear to adjust readily to these things. Others adapt less easily to the new way of life and become depressed and anxious. These feelings show in different ways. A patient may be apathetic, trying to ignore his problems. He may be agitated and aggressive. Some may even feel that life is not worth living with so many restrictions. Dialysis unit staff will offer all the support and understanding they can while the individual gradually comes to terms with his problems.

Readjustment

With the passage of time, perhaps taking years to achieve fully, the patient enters a third stage in which he is able to enjoy life whilst accepting the restrictions. This third stage probably represents a further improvement in physical health after long-term dialysis as well as a psychological adjustment. Long familiarity with dialysis techniques and with the diet makes life easier for the patient and family.

Bearing in mind the above it is easy to understand the extra difficulties that develop if any of the following occur: difficulty in developing adequate vascular access, difficulty in 'needling', reduced income or loss of a job, lack of sexual satisfaction, disruption of family life and of hobbies.

Difficulty with vascular access has been described earlier in this chapter (page 72). All that need be emphasized is that with modern surgical techniques a good fistula can eventually be made in everyone.

'Needling' may be difficult. The patient is aware that he is kept alive by use of his fistula. If the fistula is difficult to use or becomes damaged by use it may appear to threaten the person's life. This is understandable but dialysis patients do not come to permanent harm because of difficulties with their fistulae.

Dialysis takes time. The hours that have to be spent attached to a machine were used previously to earn money. For some people evening dialysis at home, or in hospital, allows them to work full-time. A few people are able to do paperwork connected with their job while on dialysis. Nevertheless many dialysis patients are unable to work full-time either because of the hours of their job or because they lack the strength for manual tasks. This may result in lower pay or unemployment. Losing a job and the need to live on social security money are frustrating to some patients. Social security benefits available for dialysis patients are covered in Chapter 19.

In general dialysis patients enjoy sex less than normal people. Men may have difficulty with erections and both men and women in renal failure are less interested in sex. Orgasms are less frequent in dialysis patients. This is bound to affect the healthy partner in addition to the more general worries about the spouse's illness and treatment. A man on dialysis may be unable to satisfy his wife or a wife on dialysis may be uninterested in relations with her husband. Unless the partner is very understanding, sexual difficulties may become very frustrating for both. This is one of the factors which have led to divorce in dialysis families. Nevertheless, divorce is less common in dialysis families than in the population in general and some marriages are strengthened as the couples support each other in overcoming their problems.

Dialysis may also affect general family life because one person has to be out of the family circle dialysing at hospital or in the dialysis room at home. Dialysis is bound to affect the family holiday and may interfere with family outings. Illness in a parent will obviously worry the children in the family.

In conclusion, dialysis treatment has to become a way of life for the patient and his family. Most renal units have a patients' society. It is a good idea to join the local group so as to meet the other patients who may be able to share useful ideas on coping with dialysis.

9

Continuous ambulatory peritoneal dialysis

Introduction and Definitions

This form of dialysis became freely available in 1980. There has been substantial increase in use of this technique, interest in the procedure and development of biomedical expertise in continuous ambulatory peritoneal dialysis (CAPD). Approximately half of all dialysis patients across the world now receive this form of treatment. Long term results are awaited but are expected to be as good as those for haemodialysis and transplantation. Because of CAPD many people are dialysed who previously would not have received treatment.

In health the kidneys continuously remove waste products and water. Haemodialysis is used for relatively short periods of time. CAPD is used every day to remove waste products and water slowly but continuously. The odd name was chosen to emphasize that the patient receiving this treatment is free to walk about, drive or work.

Some definitions are necessary:

Bacteria

This is the technical name for germs. Bacteria live normally on the skin. They do not cause disease unless the skin is broken, when they come into contact with living tissues.

Sterile

This is a common medical word which means the absence of bacteria. This is not the same use of the word which means inability to produce children. Sterile is *not* the same as clean. Clean hands, for example, will have bacteria living on them. To obtain sterile hands they must be washed for about 3 minutes and then sterile gloves (from a packet) are put on. This is the same procedure that a surgeon undertakes before starting an operation. Instruments are specially treated by heat or chemicals to sterilize them.

Antiseptic

An antiseptic is a chemical such as carbolic or iodine which can be used to destroy bacteria on the hands of an operator and the skin of a patient before any procedure is done. It reduces the number of germs present but does not remove them completely.

Aseptic

No bacteria are present under aseptic conditions. The operator wears sterile gloves, as described above, and uses sterile instruments. If the hands accidentally touch something unsterile the procedure becomes 'dirty' and the gloves must be changed.

Mask

This is a strong piece of paper about 8 × 5 inches which is placed across the nose and mouth before starting a sterile procedure. The mask is kept in place by tapes tied around the head or by elastic loops which hook over the ears. Bacteria from the nose or mouth cannot then fall onto a sterile area. In some units masks are not used during the practice of CAPD.

Peritonitis

This is infection of the peritoneum by bacteria. It is a serious illness. It results from careless technique by allowing a portion of sterile line to brush across the skin. There is pain in the belly and the dialysate which is normally clear becomes murky-white. A member of the renal unit staff must be telephoned immediately.

Dwell Time

This term refers to the length of time dialysate is allowed to stay in the abdominal cavity. For CAPD dwell time is about 6 hours.

Principle of CAPD

Dialysate is run in and left in the abdominal cavity for about 6 hours, four times each day. So that adequate dialysis is achieved the process has to be continuous but does not involve a machine. The patient dialyses himself day and night. The efficiency of the process as judged by removal of waste products is poor but the quality of life enjoyed by the patient is good. Figure 9.1 shows a comparison of the quantity of waste produced removed by haemodialysis, intermittent peritoneal dialysis and CAPD. With haemodialysis and intermittent peritoneal dialysis there is a sharp drop in the blood concentrations of waste products during the

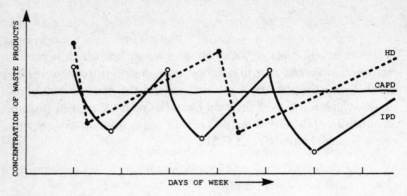

Figure 9.1 A comparison of the concentrations of waste products in the blood of three people each being treated by a different form of chronic dialysis. HD = haemodialysis; CAPD = continuous ambulatory peritoneal dialysis; IPD = intermittent peritoneal dialysis

dialysis period. In between dialyses the amount of waste products increases. With CAPD the blood concentration of these substances remains virtually constant because dialysis is continuous.

Technique of CAPD

A patient is prepared for dialysis by the insertion of a Tenckhoff catheter in the usual way (see page 54). Once the first 48 hours of rapid continuous dialysis has been finished (see page 58) CAPD is started.

The CAPD dialysis fluid comes in 2 litre (3 pint) measures in sealed plastic bags which are two-thirds full. Each bag can hold up to 3 litres (about 5 pints) so that fluid can be drained from the patient. Bags are manufactured to contain different amounts of sugar (page 55). The greater the amount of sugar the greater amount of 'suck' ('strong bags') and also the greater amount of sugar absorbed into the patient. The technique of CAPD is as follows:

(1) The bag containing 2 litres of dialysis fluid is connected to

a plastic tube (a transfer set) which in turn is connected to the end of the Tenckhoff catheter. The two connections that are made have to be done under sterile conditions. Very careful instructions are given to the patient when he trains for CAPD. The importance of the sterile technique is emphasized because there is always a risk of introducing bacteria into the line which will result in peritonitis.

(2) The bag is then hung up above the patient and the 2 litres of dialysate flow into the abdominal cavity (see Figure 9.2). The line is then clamped off.

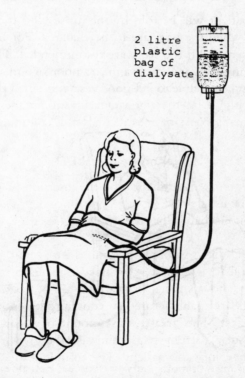

2 litre
plastic
bag of
dialysate

Figure 9.2   CAPD. 2 litres of dialysate are hung up above the patient. The fluid flows down the transfer set into the abdomen

(3) The bag is then rolled up and together with the line is tucked into the patient's pocket or placed in a pouch under the clothing.

(4) For the next 5–8 hours the patient lives normally and then prepares to change the bag for a fresh one. The first bag is unrolled and placed below the abdominal cavity so that the dialysate containing waste products and fluid from the patient runs out of the belly. This is shown in Figure 9.3. Once the dialysate has drained out of the abdomen the bag is disconnected from the line and is replaced by a fresh bag. The person then repeats steps (2)–(4).

(5) The patient will be told by the nurse who trains him the times when the bags are to be changed. For large people four cycles (8 litres) daily are recommended. This involves changing bags at about 7 a.m., 12 noon, 6 p.m. and 11 p.m. It may be possible to get good results in small people using

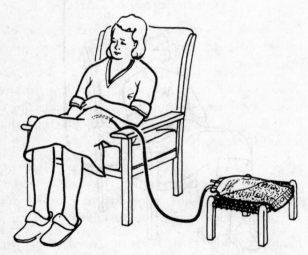

Figure 9.3   After 5 or more hours dwell time the plastic bag is unrolled and placed below the level of the patient's abdomen. Dialysate with waste products and water extracted from the patient flow out

only three cycles (6 litres) daily. For such a person the bags would need changing at approximately 7 a.m., 3 p.m. and 11 p.m.

It will be seen that CAPD, while simple, requires daily careful attention to detail.

The above system is now referred to as conventional CAPD to differentiate it from new techniques which have been developed over the past few years. The major reason for changing conventional CAPD was to reduce the chance of a patient developing bacterial peritonitis.

Whichever system is chosen one episode of peritonitis every 12 months is the maximum that should occur to any particular person. The different types of CAPD lines and bags will not be described because all a specific person requires to know is the technique used at his or her dialysis unit.

Points in Favour of CAPD

(1) *Equipment.* This system of dialysis is very simple and a patient does not have to learn to use any complicated machinery.

(2) *Training.* Two or three weeks is sufficient for anyone to master the system of connecting and disconnecting the lines from the bags. It may take months to gain the skills needed for self-haemodialysis.

(3) *Home life.* Because there is no machinery used, no modification of the patient's home is needed. Also the patient need depend very little upon a partner to help in dialysis. There is thus less strain upon the family.

(4) *Food and drinks.* CAPD patients need to eat well. The amount of fluid required may be more than a normal person needs. This is more pleasant than the small quantity of fluid allowed for the haemodialysis patient (see page 100).

(5) *Drugs.* Often only aluminium hydroxide, or calcium carbonate is needed (page 60).

(6) *Health.* A greater improvement in the anaemia of renal failure (see page 38) is seen in patients on CAPD than in those treated by haemodialysis or intermittent peritoneal dialysis. The person has more energy and is not so short of breath after physical work or sport. Figure 9.4 shows the improvement in the anaemia of renal failure in two people, one receiving haemodialysis and the other CAPD. Because the number of red blood cells is nearly doubled in CAPD patients they feel more healthy. This is a major advantage. It is believed that some waste products are better removed across the peritoneum than across the membranes of the artificial kidney (page 52). Loss of these molecules allows bone marrow to function more adequately and the haemoglobin concentration rises.

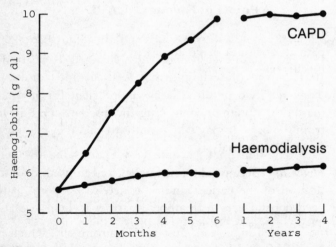

Figure 9.4 Haemoglobin plotted against time for the haemodialysis and CAPD patient. There is an early and persistent increase in the amount of haemoglobin in chronic peritoneal dialysis patients. Normal haemoglobin concentrations are more than 12 g/dl.

(7) *Travel.* CAPD dialysate is available in most European and American cities. With planning and care it is possible to travel widely whilst continuing treatment.

(8) *Diabetes.* CAPD is the best treatment for diabetics who develop permanent renal failure. Insulin is added to each bag so that the diabetes is very well controlled.

Points Against CAPD

(1) *Infections.* The risk of introducing germs into the lines and hence into the belly is considerable. Peritonitis then develops. It is painful and the patient has to return to hospital for antibiotics and more frequent dialysis cycles. Ideally peritonitis should never occur; this is so in 20% of patients.

It has been found that over time the teaching of CAPD by renal unit staff improves and shows itself by less episodes of infection.

(2) *Technique.* The person treating himself with CAPD has to be very careful each time a bag is changed. Repeating the sterile, no-touch technique may well become tedious.

(3) *Times.* The bags containing dialysate are changed three or four times daily. The run-in and run-out time together with bag changing time may add up to four or more hours each day. This may become very tedious and the person never has a day which is not partly tied up with dialysis.

(4) *Place of changing bags.* Some privacy is needed for a person to change his bag of dialysate. In addition the bag should be changed in a clean, dust-free environment, which may be difficult for the patient in full-time employment. When travelling it may be possible to use a room in the casualty department of a hospital or the medical centre of an airport in which bag changing is possible. Toilets on railways or

bus stations are unsatisfactory because adequate facilities for handwashing and clean surfaces are not guaranteed.

(5) *Sex and CAPD*. The presence of a tube entering the abdomen is off-putting to some and others think that the catheter would get in the way. Some think that the catheter makes them unattractive and believe that their partner will find it repulsive. If thought about carefully, discussed with the sexual partner and if necessary talked over with a member of the renal unit staff, there is no logical reason why a CAPD catheter should alter people's sexual habits.

(6) *Minor problems*. CAPD patients are more likely to get hernias, backache and constipation than other dialysis patients. These are not major problems but may be worrying for the person involved.

Conclusion

CAPD has expanded very rapidly since it became available. There is no doubt that it is a very satisfactory, effective, long-term treatment of kidney failure. Informed opinion now considers CAPD to be the dialysis of first choice for many people. Much effort has been made to devise easy fail-safe methods of connecting dialysate to transfer line. These efforts have been quite successful.

Many patients, previously treated with haemodialysis, who then try CAPD are very happy to remain on peritoneal dialysis. Conversely, there are some people who prefer haemodialysis to CAPD. A renal unit ideally is able to offer either form of treatment to a patient and to allow change between one type of dialysis and the other.

10

Intermittent peritoneal dialysis

Chronic intermittent peritoneal dialysis is a long-term treatment of chronic renal failure. It is less frequently used than CAPD or chronic haemodialysis but it is an established technique.

Choice of Patients for IPD

Intermittent peritoneal dialysis (IPD) is generally thought to be most suitable for three types of patients. They are:

(1) Some people for various reasons are unable to adhere to the obsessional technique necessary to practise CAPD. These people suffer recurrent episodes of peritonitis (page 79). For them IPD is more suitable.

(2) Some patients become bored with the repetitive nature of CAPD. IPD allows an escape.

(3) A few people strongly dislike the sight of their blood circulating through a dialyser and lines. IPD allows them a different form of dialysis.

Advantages of Chronic IPD

IPD is gentle in that waste products are removed much more slowly than by haemodialysis. Rapid haemodialysis often causes a patient to feel 'washed out' the day after treatment. This does not occur with IPD. The technique of IPD is easier to learn than that of haemodialysis. There is no need to gain the skill of inserting needles into a fistula (see page 50). The semi-automatic peritoneal dialysis machines available are about as complicated to set up as a haemodialysis machine but once set up are much less likely to require adjustment. 'Alarms' are less frequent and hence a dialysis is less stressful.

IPD can be used for virtually all patients except for those who previously have had a number of abdominal operations. After any operation in the abdomen the peritoneum (see page 53) becomes scarred and there is a smaller area available to act as a semi-permeable membrane (page 44). More abdominal operations mean less chance of successful peritoneal dialysis.

An important advantage of IPD is that the patient is able to drink more fluid than a patient who receives chronic haemo-dialysis. There are two reasons for this. Firstly the IPD patient treats himself two or four times each week; thus there is a shorter gap between each dialysis period compared with haemodialysis. There is therefore less time for fluid to accumulate between dialyses. Secondly, because the dialysis period is long (see next section) the patient is able to drink whilst on dialysis and the fluid is removed shortly after it has been taken.

Disadvantages of IPD

There are three main disadvantages:

(1) *Length of dialysis*. IPD is slow. About 36–48 hours of dialysis each week are necessary. This period is split into two to four periods and is restricting.

(2) *The Tenckhoff catheter*. The position of this catheter in the

belly has been described in Chapter 5. It is not uncomfortable but it is inconvenient whilst bathing. It makes sun-
bathing embarrassing and is sexually inhibiting.

(3) *Need for a suitable room.* Intermittent peritoneal dialysis
requires a room or cabin set aside specifically for the
machine just as for home haemodialysis. There is even less
chance of hospital IPD than hospital haemodialysis because
of the long periods of time needed for dialysis. The setting
up of a dialysis room at home is assisted by the Home
Dialysis Administrator. This is fully described in Chapter
14.

Technique of IPD

A few definitions are necessary to make this section clear.

Inflow Time

This is the time taken for the peritoneal dialysis fluid (dialysate)
to flow from the machine into the patient's abdomen via the lines
and Tenckhoff catheter. An average inflow time is about 4 to 5
minutes but varies with the rate at which the machine pumps the
fluid and the size of the patient's abdominal cavity. A large man
may require a longer inflow time than a small woman. It is
important to know the inflow time because this is one of the
adjustments that a patient may need to make to his machine.

Dwell Time

This is the period for which dialysate remains within the abdomen.
Waste products pass from blood vessels in the peritoneum into
the dialysate. This is peritoneal dialysis – see page 52. Generally
dwell time for IPD patients is about 15 to 20 minutes but may
vary. Like the inflow time the length of the dwell time can be
changed by adjusting the machine.

Outflow Time

The outflow time is the number of minutes taken for the dialysate to flow out of the abdominal cavity. It is usually about 15–20 minutes and can be altered by adjusting the machine. It may be necessary to adjust the outflow time more frequently than either the inflow or dwell times.

Cycle Time

This is the total time taken by inflow, dwell and outflow times. From the above figures a cycle lasts about 35–40 minutes. If dialysate flows very freely in and out of the catheter it may be possible to complete two cycles each hour. Rapid cycle times are good because the efficiency of the peritoneal dialysis is improved and this leads to shorter total hours per week.

Patient Line

This is the sterile plastic tube which runs from the machine and is connected to the Tenckhoff catheter. Dialysate runs from the machine via the patient line to the abdominal cavity and after the dwell period back via the patient line through the machine to the drains.

Procedure for automated IPD

This section only covers the technique in broad outline. Figure 10.1 outlines an IPD machine connected to a patient. Details of procedure vary in different units and a patient being taught IPD would receive precise instructions in his particular unit. The procedure may be broken down into the following steps:

(1) The patient weighs himself and takes his blood pressure lying and standing.

(2) The machine is switched on and the dialysis parameters are set (inflow time, dwell time, number of cycles).

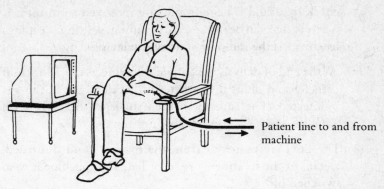

Patient line to and from machine

Figure 10.1 A diagram of a person receiving treatment from a semi-automatic intermittent peritoneal dialysis machine. Dialysate flows into and out of the patient's abdomen via the patient line as shown by the arrows

(3) The patient attaches the various lines to the machine and connects them to the dialysis storage containers.

(4) Next, after carefully washing hands and perhaps wearing a mask and sterile gloves, the patient undoes and swabs the free end of the Tenckhoff catheter with antiseptic solution. Then the Tenckhoff catheter is attached to the patient line from the machine. It is difficult to explain how this is done – the procedure can only be learnt by practice. It is however essential that these steps are done exactly as taught because there is a risk of introducing germs into the patient's abdominal cavity and hence causing an infection (peritonitis).

(5) The patient commences treatment. Provided that the machine is correctly adjusted and working properly there is little to do for the next 12 to 20 or so hours.

(6) During this time the blood pressure must be measured a few times and the patient may need to weigh himself to

check that fluid is being gradually removed from him. It is a time that can be occupied by reading, writing, sleeping, listening to the radio or watching television.

(7) At the end of dialysis the patient disconnects the Tenckhoff catheter and plugs the catheter off, taking care not to get it infected. The catheter is then stuck to the belly with adhesive tape in a comfortable position.

(8) The lines are removed from the machine and discarded. Details of the treatment are recorded. The machine is then switched off.

(9) At about the same time the patient weighs himself and again measures his blood pressure lying and standing. The dialysis is now completed. The average weight loss is 1–2 kg during each dialysis.

Conclusion

The use of IPD is not widespread. There are considerably more people receiving CAPD than IPD. Nevertheless if correctly chosen and carefully used IPD gives a patient good dialyses and satisfactory quality of life.

11

Continuous cycle peritoneal dialysis

This form of dialysis works on exactly the same principle as all forms of peritoneal dialysis (page 52). It was developed from CAPD and IPD. Continuous cycle peritoneal dialysis (CCPD) is less frequently used than CAPD but is a very satisfactory treatment.

Choice of Patients for CCPD

Continuous cycle peritoneal dialysis is used for similar reasons as IPD described in the previous chapter (page 87). Some people find it more convenient to dialyse themselves for 8–10 hours over night than to perform CAPD (page 79) or to spend rather long periods on IPD (page 88).

Advantages of CCPD

These are very similar to those of intermittent peritoneal dialysis.

(1) The treatment is gentle and the technique easy to learn.

(2) Like CAPD and IPD, fluid and diet allowances are more generous than for the patient receiving haemodialysis. The gap between each CCPD treatment is approximately 14 hours.

(3) An important advantage is that the patient is able to treat himself at home without the help of a partner.

(4) The machine used is considerably smaller than that necessary for IPD and requires little space. Virtually any bedroom is large enough to accommodate a CCPD machine. It has wheels and can be pushed into a cupboard during the day.

(5) It follows that little or no modification of a patient's home is required to perform CCPD.

(6) If set up correctly the chance of peritonitis (page 79) is very small. Some people have treated themselves for more than 4 years without peritoneal infection.

Disadvantages of CCPD

(1) This is a slow treatment and the fact that it is performed every night proves irksome for some people.

(2) A chronic peritoneal dialysis catheter is necessary with its associated disadvantages – infection (page 79), bathing and others (pages 39 and 86).

Procedure for CCPD

Only an outline of the technique will be given. Any person planning CCPD treatment will be taught the technique of the unit in question. Details differ from one dialysis unit to another and to some extent are modified to suit a particular person's needs. The following is an outline:

(1) The machine is plugged into the mains electricity supply and switched on.

(2) A large bag, or smaller bags, of dialysis fluid is placed on a drip stand which is part of the CCPD machine.

(3) The apparatus is then programmed to allow four cycles, each of 2 litres to run into the patient's abdomen over the course of the next 10 hours.

(4) The patient weighs himself and takes his blood pressure.

(5) Under aseptic conditions the Tenckhoff catheter is attached to the patient line. This must be done with care because of the risk of introducing germs into dialysate and hence the abdominal cavity. Nevertheless, compared with CAPD this has to be performed only once a day.

(6) At this stage, usually towards the end of the evening, the patient presses a button to set the machine into the dialysis mode.

(7) A CCPD machine is very safe and simple so that patients can sleep with the confidence that warmed dialysate will automatically be run into their abdominal cavity, dwell for $2\frac{1}{2}$ hours, be allowed to run out, volume checked by measuring its weight and a further 2 litres run in.

(8) At the end of the dialysis period the patient disconnects his Tenckhoff catheter from the patient line, weighs himself and measures his blood pressure.

(9) He is then free to go about his daily activities.

Conclusion

Continuous cycle peritoneal dialysis has been available for approximately 5 years. It is used less commonly than CAPD although this may change. Some machines can be taken apart and transported in the boot of a car for holidays. Further, like arrangements for CAPD fluid, machines and CCPD fluid are available throughout the developed world allowing holidays to be taken much further afield.

12

Diet and renal failure

Introduction

Nowadays the word 'diet' most commonly refers to a scheme for slimming. However, in some diseases, including kidney disease, special diets are prescribed. The aim is to advise the patient what foods he may eat in what quantities to maintain him in the best possible health. The kind of diet advised for a renal patient will depend on the severity of the illness and the type of treatment being given.

So as not to lead to confusion only the bare outlines will be described. Every renal unit has an associated dietician who has special experience with renal diets. Each patient receives specific and practical advice about foods that are suitable and about those that must not be eaten or should be restricted. In addition the dietician will help in suggesting recipes which sometimes may be useful for a patient with particular dietetic needs. As far as possible each diet is tailored to a patient's particular need to fit in with dietary preferences and cultural background. Special recipes can be devised to increase the variety of the diet.

Diets for Patients with Advanced Chronic Renal Failure

The aim of a diet here is to provide the best possible nutrition which will help to improve health, given that the patient has chronic kidney failure. The specific aims of a diet recommended by a dietician are as follows:

(1) To obtain a balance of protein, energy, vitamins and minerals.

(2) To reduce the amount of waste products accumulating in the blood. During the 1980s it has been realized that reduction in the amount of protein in the diet may slow the rate of development of terminal renal failure. By this dietary treatment it may be possible to put off the time for starting dialysis for a year or more. As yet it is not known whether some patients may respond to a reduced protein diet better than others. This important topic is being studied in many countries. A renal dietician has the skill to provide the information for a reduced protein diet which is adjusted to the patients' likes and dislikes. Generally about 35 g of protein daily is suggested but this varies according to the size and occupation of the particular patient.

(3) Before dialysis is started some people lose their appetite and may feel sick. Here again a dietician is able to help.

On a diet sheet the weight of foods is expressed in ounces or grams. The relationship is 1 oz = 30 g. For simplicity some equate 1 oz with 25 g because this makes the arithmetic easier and does not cause great errors.

The diet alone is often all that is needed. Some doctors prescribe aluminium hydroxide or calcium carbonate at this stage. This has been discussed on page 60. Occasionally salt capsules or vitamin tablets are prescribed. The reason for giving them would be explained to the patient.

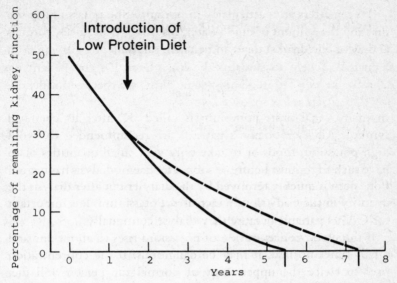

Figure 12.1 This diagram shows what is thought to happen if a person begins a strict low protein diet years before terminal renal failure occurs compared with the expected rate of decline of function if normal food was eaten. It appears likely that the low protein diet slows the rate of loss of filtering ability of the kidneys so that the patient may not require dialysis for more than one year longer had standard food been eaten. This is beneficial to all concerned

Haemodialysis Diets

Once a person is on dialysis the protein content of the diet is increased to approximately normal. This amount varies from unit to unit and patient to patient. The dietician often visits dialysis wards to talk to patients about the best foods for health. For example, advice on the correct proportions of animal protein (meat, fish, cheese, milk, eggs) and vegetable protein (bread, cereal, rice, potatoes) in relation to ample calories is important. For diabetics and vegetarians special help is available.

Two matters are particularly important – the potassium in the diet and the amount of fluid (water, tea, soup, fruit juices, cordials and alcoholic drinks) that can be taken safely.

Potassium

In many renal units potassium is called 'K' after its chemical symbol. All haemodialysis patients are recommended to avoid high potassium foods or to take only very small quantities or to have such a food just before or soon after haemodialysis has begun. Potassium is quickly removed by the dialyser but after dialysis the quantity in the body slowly increases. Potassium is less important for CAPD patients because they dialyse continually.

If the blood concentration of potassium rises to about one and a half times normal, it may be dangerous. If the concentration rises to twice the upper limit of normal the person will die. Probably a number of dialysis patients have killed themselves by taking too much potassium. High potassium is dangerous because it alters the rhythm of the heart which eventually painlessly stops.

A brief list of high potassium foods is given in Table 12.1.

Fluid Intake

Most people on dialysis find that they produce less urine after a few weeks of treatment. Water is removed during dialysis by ultrafiltration (see pages 50 and 55) but in between dialyses only one or two cupfuls of urine are made each day. This means that the haemodialysis patient should not drink more than about a pint of fluid daily. Drinking more than this cannot 'force' the kidneys to get rid of the excess. The extra fluid remains in the body and the pre-dialysis weight (described on page 68) will be too high. During dialysis additional ultrafiltration will be needed which may be unpleasant.

If a patient has been foolish and drunk much more fluid than is safe the extra fluid can accumulate in the lungs. This may only

Table 12.1 High potassium foods. This is only a short list; the advice of the dietician should be asked for other foods. With assistance from your dietician some may be eaten at times

Fruits	Vegetables
Avocado	Jerusalem Artichoke
Apricots	Dried vegetables – haricot,
Bananas	kidney and soya beans, chick
Dried fruit – currants, dates,	peas
figs, prunes	Mushrooms
Kiwi fruit	Potatoes – baked, chips, roast
Passion fruit	Spinach
Pomegranate	
Rhubarb	
Nuts and snacks	*Fluids*
All nuts	Beer or cider
Peanut butter	Chocolate drinks
Marzipan	Evaporated and condensed milk
Crisps	Instant coffee
Chocolate	Juice from tinned fruits
Fruit gums	Sweet wines
Liquorice	

cause increased shortness of breath before dialysis but could be very unpleasant or even fatal.

Reduction of fluid intake for a haemodialysis patient may prove to be the most difficult restriction with this type of treatment. With practice and help from staff of the renal unit, patients are able to manage so that their pre-dialysis weight is not more than 2 kg above their 'dry' weight post-dialysis. Fluid restriction is more difficult in hot weather, and for those who receive haemodialysis twice weekly rather than three times a week. A common error is to forget that *all* fluid foods have to be counted in the daily allowance. This must be remembered when custard, gravy, ice cream, ice cubes, jelly, soup or yoghurt are taken. It is also worth noting that salty foods make a person more thirsty.

If fluid restriction becomes irksome some of the following may be of help:

Limit yourself to a small amount of fluid at set times.

Use a smaller cup.

Rinse the mouth with water and *spit* it out.

Suck a boiled sweet or chew gum.

Suck a slice of lemon.

Suck ice cubes but do not swallow the water when melted.

Continuous Ambulatory Peritoneal Dialysis Diets

Eating correct foods is important for CAPD patients but the restrictions are different from those for haemodialysis patients. The single most obvious advantage of CAPD is that the amount of fluid taken over a 24 hour period is 1000 to 1200 ml (up to 2 pints). Nevertheless because CAPD dialysate contains sugar (page 55) which is absorbed, a patient may easily put on weight (fat) if some restriction of energy foods is not practised. When a person begins CAPD the following general points will be explained by the dietician.

(1) The protein intake is raised to normal for the person's size and age and sufficient to compensate for blood protein that passes into dialysate.

(2) Sugars and fats must be controlled because of the tendency to put on weight.

(3) Some salt restriction may be needed to reduce thirst and perhaps to lower high blood pressure.

(4) The amount of potassium eaten may need to be reduced if the concentration of potassium in the blood becomes too high.

(5) Fibre intake – for example wholegrain cereals, wholemeal bread and bran should be high because such foods help avoid constipation to which CAPD patients are prone.

(6) The attraction of less fluid restriction than for a haemo-dialysis patient has been mentioned above. A comparison of fluids that may be safely taken for patients receiving different treatments of chronic renal failure is shown in Table 12.2.

Intermittent Peritoneal Dialysis Diets

Peritoneal dialysis is a slow process, the average patient requiring 36–48 hours treatment each week. The treatment periods are usually about 15–20 hours long (see page 88). Peritoneal dialysis removes water from the patient whilst dialysis proceeds. Some blood protein is lost into the dialysate; the patient must therefore eat sufficient protein so that he does not become undernourished.

Between dialysis periods restrictions similar to those for the haemodialysis patient apply.

Diet After Transplantation

One of the pleasant features of a successful transplant is that the person concerned can have a meal of his choice and perhaps eat some foods which previously have had to be restricted.

Nevertheless it is sensible to eat a balanced diet to help maintain the best health. Thus a person with a transplant kidney should choose his foods with the following in mind:

(1) Avoid an excess of sugar and very sweet foods.

(2) Do not eat much animal fat; polyunsaturated fats are healthier.

Table 12.2 A comparison of food and fluid for patients with severe renal disease receiving different treatments

	Protein	Salt	Potassium	Phosphate	Fluids
Chronic renal failure	restricted	usually normal	usually normal	restricted	usually normal
Haemodialysis	virtually normal	restricted: salt in cooking only	restricted: avoid high potassium foods	restricted	very restricted
Chronic peritoneal dialysis	normal	may need to be restricted	normal or some restriction	some restriction	some restriction
Transplantation	normal	normal	normal	normal	normal

(3) A high fibre diet makes good sense. Thus wholemeal bread, wholegrain cereals, beans and peas (pulses) should be eaten regularly.

(4) Too much salt in cooking, at the table or salt preserved foods (such as bacon, ham, cheese, ham, pate, salted fish or sausages) should be avoided.

Again the renal dietician is able to help with these matters. The above suggestions relate not only to transplant recipients but to the whole population.

Conclusion

Different stages and different treatments of renal failure require different food and fluid intakes. Advice from a dietician is essential to gain the best quality health. All renal diets are modified to suit the preferences of the particular patient.

13

Fertility, pregnancy and contraception

It is well known that some people with renal failure have sexual difficulties (page 39). It is often forgotten that female patients may be fertile. In addition fertility changes according to the type of treatment. As a woman develops progressive renal failure her periods and ovulation (egg shedding) may become irregular. Some periods occur without ovulation.

Haemodialysis

When on haemodialysis perhaps half of women remain fertile despite irregular or no periods. It is therefore possible that they may conceive. It is very unlikely that a pregnancy will continue for the usual 40 weeks. There are perhaps only 20 to 30 babies worldwide born to women on haemodialysis. The majority of such pregnancies end in a spontaneous abortion at 12 to 16 weeks.

Because it cannot easily be determined which women on haemodialysis are fertile and those who are not it is prudent that all avoid pregnancy. Generally a condom (sheath) or a diaphragm (cap) is recommended. For the woman who has completed her family sterilisation or vasectomy of her husband is advisable.

Chronic Peritoneal Dialysis

Women of childbearing years receiving CAPD or CCPD are likely to be more fertile than those on haemodialysis. Precautions must be more stringent.

Transplantation

After a woman has received a transplant kidney which functions well, normal menstruation and fertility return. With health improving at the same time, sexual activity is likely to increase and thus the chance of pregnancy rises.

If a woman at this stage plans a pregnancy she should probably wait for about 12 months until the function of the new kidney is known to be stable. Such pregnancies are usually safe for both mother and child but delivery tends to be premature. Neither pregnancy nor delivery adversely affect the function of the transplant kidney. Nevertheless before becoming pregnant it is sensible for the woman to discuss matters with her renal physician and perhaps also an obstetrician.

For those women who do not want children contraception will be required. A coil should not be used because of the risk of infection. Usually one of the other conventional methods proves satisfactory.

14

Home dialysis

Home dialysis means that a patient dialyses himself at home without any direct help or supervision from his renal unit.

Home dialysis usually means home haemodialysis but there are some people at home treating themselves with CCPD or IPD. There are a large number of people using CAPD which is exclusively a home dialysis technique. This chapter is written primarily for the home haemodialysis patient but some of the general points may be useful for people on CAPD, CCPD or home intermittent peritoneal dialysis.

Selection of Patients for Home Haemodialysis

Home dialysis is the preferred form of treatment for long-term haemodialysis. If all patients remained on hospital dialysis there would be no room to take on new patients just starting dialysis.

All major renal units have patients on home dialysis. The plan of treatment may vary from unit to unit. For example:

(1) Home dialysis for one year after which the patient may choose to go on the waiting list for a transplant.

(2) Home dialysis for those not interested in a transplant, at least not at first.

(3) Home dialysis for those in whom a renal transplant has failed, whilst awaiting another.

Not every home is suitable for home dialysis as it stands. If there is a spare room additional plumbing and wiring can be laid on. A cabin could be erected in the garden if there is no spare room. In some cases it may be necessary to move house although in these circumstances CAPD or CCPD would be advised for simplicity and economy.

Every renal unit with home dialysis patients has a member of staff called the Home Dialysis Administrator. He or she is not necessarily qualified in nursing but is experienced in dialysis and advises about the suitability of a particular home for dialysis and the adaptations or extension which may be needed. He also assesses what alterations to water and electricity supplies will be required. Subsequently the Home Dialysis Administrator is responsible for the regular delivery of stores and acts as a link between the patient and the renal unit staff. The cost of home modification, electricity, installation and rent of a telephone or extension to a pre-existing telephone is borne by the hospital concerned.

Most renal units have a printed sheet of advice and instructions for potential home dialysis patients. Advice by telephone is always available.

Suitability for Home Haemodialysis

Self treatment appears daunting at first sight. In fact, given time, good training and sufficient practice to gain confidence and expertise virtually anybody can master the skills necessary to dialyse himself. Much depends upon the motivation of the patient: if he believes that he will succeed time and training will prove him to be correct. He must be willing to accept considerable responsibility for his own treatment and to undertake some hours of work on his own behalf each week. Successful home dialysis does not depend so much upon the intelligence or dexterity of the person as upon his will to succeed. The full support and co-operation of a spouse or close family member is essential.

Intermittent peritoneal dialysis technique is easier to learn than haemodialysis, but peritoneal dialysis is more time-consuming (see page 88). CAPD is very easy to learn but is also time-consuming.

Training of the Home Haemodialysis Patient

Training takes at least two months. Should a patient fall ill or should technical difficulties develop, training will be prolonged. Often the time of starting dialysis at home is determined by the time taken to modify the patient's home for dialysis. If rehousing is necessary it may take many months.

During the training period the patient must learn in detail about dialysis, care of fistulae, technical procedures such as the sterilization and washing of the dialyser, diet, measurement of pulse and blood pressure and how to deal with emergencies whilst on dialysis. In addition the patient must learn most of the technical terms concerned with dialysis (more than are included in this book). Should some difficulty develop whilst a patient is dialysing at home he can ring his renal unit staff and discuss what to do in precise terms.

During the last few weeks of training the patient's spouse, partner or some reliable adult will come to the dialysis unit with the patient to be trained to help the patient in needling and other procedures necessary for dialysis.

Most of the training will be given by one nurse – the Home Dialysis Sister. Later when the patient is at home the sister will visit and will help with advice by telephone. Her visits are in addition to those of the Home Dialysis Administrator.

The patient will probably use the same machine at home which he has used in training. Thus any minor peculiarities of the equipment will already be familiar to him. In addition the patient will use during training the same type of dialyser that he will afterwards use at home.

Equipment Required

As described a spare room is modified or a cabin is placed in the garden. A de-ionizer is put between the main water tank and the inlet to the kidney machine to remove excess calcium from 'hard' water.

The kidney machine together with a supply of dialysers, lines, needles and smaller items is delivered to the patient's home. A telephone extension is essential to the dialysis room. The telephone is given priority by British Telecom for repair should it break down.

Dialysate concentrate is delivered by the manufacturers. The dialysis machine is serviced by the renal unit technicians or in some cases by the manufacturers. The Home Dialysis Administrator will arrange with the local council to collect used dialysis lines, needles and dialysers, for disposal.

Advantages of Home Dialysis

Most home dialysis patients agree that the major advantage of self treatment is the independence that they gain. They avoid travelling to hospital and become less of a 'patient' and more a private individual. Dialysis times can be made more flexible and thus fit in better with family and social life. Home dialysis patients tend to be fitter than their hospital counterparts. Many home dialysis patients often say that they would have started dialysing at home sooner if they had appreciated the advantages.

In Great Britain there are more people on home dialysis compared with hospital dialysis than in any country in the world. From the point of view of the Department of Health home haemodialysis is more economical than hospital haemodialysis. The costs per year have been estimated at up to £15,000 for home haemodialysis and £20,000 for hospital haemodialysis (1987 prices).

Difficulties with Home Dialysis

Problems may be technical or psychological.

Technical Problems

The commonest technical problem is difficulty with the insertion of the dialysis needles. This snag usually occurs within the first few weeks of treatment at home. The change from hospital to home dialysis naturally makes the patient nervous at first. Unless he is fully confident of the 'needling' technique he may well fail to insert the needles properly sometimes. If not successful at the first attempt, confidence ebbs and subsequent attempts become progressively less likely to be successful. No one should try to 'needle' himself more than four or five times at one go. If there is difficulty the patient should ring up his renal unit. One of four suggestions will be made:

(1) To come to the unit so that the fistula can be examined, the needles inserted and a hospital dialysis be carried out.

(2) To have the needles put in at the unit, then to return home to dialyse.

(3) To rest the arm so that the bruising will diminish and the patient can try again the next day.

(4) For a member of the renal unit staff to go to the patient's home and insert the needles.

The Home Dialysis Sister will be at the patient's home to provide moral support for the beginning of the first few dialyses. Difficulties with 'needling' may however occur a month or so after home dialysis has started.

Once a patient has passed through the stage of difficulty with 'needling' the only technical problems are likely to be defects in the kidney machine or water softener. These do not happen often.

Psychological Problems

These have been discussed on pages 39–40, 76 and 86. The home dialysis patient has probably largely adjusted to these by the time he is established at home. But the very fact that a patient is treating himself at home raises one further problem for some people. The dialysis equipment is in the home and the patient's disability is brought more obviously and continually to his notice. The hospital dialysis patient can try to put the dialysis side of his life behind him when he is not at the hospital, leaving the responsibility to someone else. The home dialysis patient cannot do this. It may seem to him and to his family that the household revolves round the dialysis room. In most homes eventually it becomes accepted as part of the day-to-day routine. There are however a few patients and their partners who find home haemodialysis a greater strain than they had anticipated, and have to give up the attempt. In this event CAPD may prove to be a satisfactory treatment. It has the advantage that no equipment is required in the patient's home. CCPD could be used if CAPD proved unsatisfactory.

15

Dialysis and holidays

Most families look forward to, enjoy and need a week or two away from home each year. Many British families in the last decade have become used to a regular holiday on some sunny beach. If one of the family is receiving regular haemodialysis treatment he becomes very limited by the number of days that are free from dialysis.

Haemodialysis

A hospital haemodialysis patient is usually dialysed twice weekly. This gives two gaps of two and three days between dialyses. A home haemodialysis patient usually dialyses three times weekly. There are therefore two gaps of one day and one of two days. It is difficult for the haemodialysis patient to fit in even a short break. The gap between dialyses can be lengthened occasionally to five days but this may be hazardous and towards the end of the five-day period the patient may feel unwell.

If the haemodialysis patient is to go on holiday he must either take equipment with him or go to a place where there are dialysis machines. Over the past decade a number of centres have been developed throughout Europe which contain holiday accommodation and haemodialysis facilities. In America the same is true.

There are a few portable dialysis machines – the best known is the Redy system. This machine weighs 65 lbs (30 kg) and can be put in the boot of a car. It does not require a continuous supply of water unlike most machines and is used with a disposable dialyser. All that is needed is $5\frac{1}{2}$ litres of water and mains electricity supply. The Redy system has proved very useful for haemodialysis patients on holiday and also for some patients who have to travel for business purposes. However the Redy dialysis system uses expensive disposable equipment.

The patients of a number of renal units have raised money to buy a communal holiday chalet which has accommodation and cooking facilities for the family and an area equipped for dialysis. Each dialysis family is able to rent the chalet from the kidney patients' association of the hospital and holiday in it for a period during the summer months. The disadvantage of a chalet is that the renal unit patients have to take their holidays in the same place year after year. The Redy system allows greater freedom of choice for a holiday.

Hospital haemodialysis patients tend not to be able to use the holiday facilities described above because they may not be able to dialyse themselves without supervision. Unfortunately in Britain patients of one renal unit are not generally welcomed for temporary dialysis in another renal unit in a holiday area. This is for two reasons. Most dialysis units have a tight schedule in dialysing their own patients which leaves little time or room for visitors. Secondly there is a chance that hepatitis could be transmitted by a patient from a unit where the hepatitis virus is present and infect staff or patients in the host unit. Nevertheless lists are available of those units in different parts of the world which are able to accommodate patients requiring haemodialysis whilst on holiday or business.

Peritoneal Dialysis

Patients receiving chronic peritoneal dialysis are much more free to go on holiday or away for a weekend than are those on haemodialysis. CAPD dialysate is available worldwide (page 85). Some CCPD machines are portable in a car boot. Machine dialysate can be obtained in many cities of the world (page 96). For a three day weekend 24 litres (8 × 3) of CAPD dialysate can be carried in a car.

Practical Matters

If planning a holiday or business trip abroad, a dialysis patient should consider the following:

(1) Have adequate insurance.

(2) Take a good supply of drugs and disposable items of equipment. Both may be difficult to obtain at short notice when abroad.

(3) Obtain a letter from the dialysis sister containing details of treatment. A similar letter from the renal physician concerning diagnosis and specific drug therapy may be useful.

(4) If visiting EEC countries obtain form E111, from the local Social Security Office. You will then be able to reclaim much of the costs of treatment in EEC countries which have reciprocal agreements with Britain.

16

Transplantation

Introduction and Definitions

There are two forms of treatment for chronic renal failure –
dialysis and kidney transplantation. No individual is committed
indefinitely to one or other form of treatment. Every renal unit
has a flexible policy which offers to each patient treatment best
suited to the stage reached in his illness. Every person who wishes
to have a transplant will need dialysis to keep him alive until a
suitable kidney becomes available. If, at some time after transplantation, the new kidney fails, the patient then goes back to
haemodialysis or peritoneal dialysis. There are some people who
have received three or four transplant kidneys. A patient may
never wish to receive a transplant kidney. For him the best
treatment would be home haemodialysis or CAPD.

A person does not have to decide, therefore, that he or she will
have to stick to one or other type of treatment. Different treatments are used at different times, taking into account the wishes
and needs of the individual.

A few terms need defining to make this chapter clear.

Transplantation or *grafting* is the operation of putting a kidney obtained from another person, known as the donor, into a patient known as the recipient. The kidney is known as the graft kidney.

Donor kidneys are of two types, live and cadaver. A live donor kidney is obtained from an identical twin, brother, sister, parent or perhaps a cousin of the patient. A cadaver kidney is rapidly removed from a person who has just died. Cadaver kidneys are most frequently used.

Rejection. Normally the human body cannot accept tissues from a different individual except in the special case of identical twins. Rejection is the process by which the body destroys transplanted organs. Continuous treatment with drugs is necessary to enable the recipient to tolerate the graft kidney. In spite of drugs, rejection may occur. There are two main forms – acute rejection and chronic rejection.

Acute rejection occurs most frequently in the first three months after a transplant operation. The graft kidney rapidly begins to fail over a period of hours. Acute rejection also occurs if the patient does not take anti-rejection drugs for a few days.

Chronic rejection is a slow process of graft kidney failure occurring over months or years.

Drugs. There are three main drugs used after transplantation: prednisolone (a form of cortisone) azathioprine (trade name Imuran) and cyclosporin. These compounds work in different ways and are used in combination to diminish or prevent rejection of the graft kidney.

Blood Groups. There are four main blood groups: O, A, B and AB. Groups O and A are the commonest. Group B is uncommon and only about 3 per cent of the population have the AB blood group. The blood group is important in transplantation because the donor must be of a blood group which can be accepted by the recipient. In principle, the matching of blood groups is similar to the matching which is necessary for blood transfusions.

Tissue typing. In addition to a specific blood group, each individual has a combination of about six main tissue types. Before grafting an attempt may be made to match the tissue types of the donor and recipient.

Points For and Against Kidney Transplantation

There is as yet no ideal form of treatment for people with chronic renal failure. In this section the pros and cons of kidney transplantation are set out.

The Advantages of Transplantation

The greatest advantage of a successful transplant is freedom. There is release from repeated and perhaps boring, unpleasant dialyses. No longer does the patient have to stick to drinking a small quantity of fluid each day. His diet is no longer restricted. It is possible to go on holiday without making complicated plans or to return home or to hospital after a few days for dialysis. For women, periods return to normal and they become capable of bearing children again. For men, potency returns and a normal sexual life is possible.

After a successful transplant, a person feels healthier because anaemia and related chronic tiredness disappear. Full-time work may not be possible when on dialysis, but should be possible after a transplant. There is an unequivocal improvement in quality of life.

The Disadvantages of Transplantation

An anaesthetic and an operation are necessary. The operation takes about four hours and might be classified as being in the 'medium major' class.

Before the transplant operation it may be necessary to undergo other operations to prepare for the transplant surgery. These might include the removal of the diseased kidneys or surgery to the bladder.

Before operation it must be recognized that the transplanted kidney might never work. The donor kidney would have to be removed, and the patient would then return to chronic dialysis to wait for the next suitable kidney. Some transplanted kidneys gradually lose their function and the patient returns to chronic dialysis.

A minor disadvantage is the need to take drugs every day without fail to prevent rejection as long as the graft lasts.

This is only a brief discussion of the advantages and disadvantages of kidney transplantation. The choice is for the patient to make in consultation with doctors.

Side Effects of Anti-rejection Drugs

Everyone who receives a transplant kidney must take drugs each day to prevent rejection. There are three main drugs each of which has different side effects.

For many years the only drugs were prednisolone and azathioprine which were taken together.

Azathioprine (Imuran) is a yellow tablet containing 50 mg of drug. An average dose is 2 to 4 tablets daily, the precise dose is decided individually for each kidney recipient. Used correctly azathioprine is very safe. The only side effect that matters is a reduction in the number of white cells produced by the bone marrow if the dose is too high. This effect is overcome by reducing the dose.

Prednisolone. These are white tablets and have many possible side effects at times described in medical articles in the lay press, which can cause anxiety for people advised by their doctors to take prednisolone. The most common effects are:

(1) Prednisolone stimulates the appetite so that unless care is taken marked weight gain occurs.

(2) Daily doses of prednisolone lead to the collection of abnormal amounts of salt and water in the body. This has two effects: firstly a tendency to raise blood pressure and secondly some

swelling of the ankles. Both can be treated with other drugs but this means taking yet more tablets.

(3) The round 'moon' face which develops after some weeks of treatment is well known.

(4) If prednisolone is taken at a prolonged high dose there is an increased chance of developing an infection. At a dose of 10 mg daily the increased chance is very small.

(5) Long term prednisolone may lead to the development of diabetes.

(6) After some years of treatment bones become weaker than normal (osteoporosis). In particular the hip joint is affected.

(7) Stretch marks on the skin of trunk and thighs are a measure of prednisolone damage to the tissues of the skin.

It may appear strange that prednisolone and other cortisone-related drugs are so widely used. The reason is straightforward: no other drug has the power to suppress rejection and immune diseases. The useful actions of prednisolone must be balanced against the possible side effects. If a person wants a transplant kidney, it must be accepted that some of the side effects of the drug may occur. This was true until cyclosporin became freely available in 1983.

Cyclosporin is a liquid with an unpleasant taste. It is taken once or twice a day with either milk or orange juice from a china cup or a glass. If mixed in plastic containers some of the drug sticks to the plastic and the patient receives too little of the dose. Cyclosporin is a powerful drug which much reduces the chances of acute rejection. Nearly all transplant centres are now using cyclosporin and results have improved. There are two main side effects which occur if the dose is too high.

(1) The liver may be injured.

(2) Kidney function may be damaged.

In either case the dose is reduced and improvement occurs. The amount of cyclosporin required varies from person to person and is judged by measuring the amount remaining in the blood approximately 12 hours after the last dose.

Currently prednisolone and azathioprine used for anti-rejection therapy are referred to as 'conventional therapy' while cyclosporin is referred to by name. Apart from the fact that cyclosporin is a powerful drug, the great advantage is that it can be used without prednisolone. Usually cyclosporin and prednisolone are combined for the first 3 to 6 months after a transplant and then prednisolone is gradually reduced and stopped. In this manner long term side effects of prednisolone are avoided.

Deciding Whether to Have a Kidney Transplant

Several points need to be considered.

Age. Young people tolerate operations better than old people. Transplantation is therefore more appropriate for patients aged between 15 and 60 years. Nevertheless, successful grafting has been performed in people over 65.

Physical fitness. Other than renal failure the person should be fit.

Living alone. Long-term haemodialysis is best conducted at home or in a minimal care dialysis centre. Ideally a single person does not dialyse himself alone in his home because of the lack of help if a serious problem develops. Unfortunately, there are few minimal care dialysis centres in Britain. Generally, therefore, a graft kidney is preferred for the patient who has no close relatives.

Impossibility of home dialysis. It may be impossible to arrange home dialysis for every individual. The home may be too small to set aside a room for dialysis; the water supply may be inadequate; moving to a bigger house may not be practical or the person may lack confidence in self-dialysis technique. CAPD may prove impossible or unacceptable in some people. In these circumstances, a transplant operation may be the way to avoid long-term dialysis in hospital or CAPD.

Need for freedom. Long-term peritoneal and haemodialysis are time-consuming. Perhaps twenty-five hours of each week are spent in preparing, dialysing and cleaning up afterwards. Intermittent peritoneal dialysis takes even more time. Chronic ambulatory peritoneal dialysis is a daily chore. A successful graft kidney will allow greater freedom.

Boredom with dialysis. Some people become bored with the unending chores of dialysis and whilst in good health feel the need for a different form of treatment. After a number of years of home dialysis or CAPD this is understandable and is a good reason for asking for a graft kidney.

Difficulties with dialysis. Some people are unable to come to terms with the restrictions which have to be placed upon them for dialysis. For the occasional patient, haemodialysis may be technically difficult each time. For such a person, a transplant kidney is a solution to his difficulties.

The prospective transplant patient and his doctors should discuss all these aspects thoroughly before a decision is reached.

Waiting List for Transplantation

When a patient has decided to have a transplant his name, details of his blood group and tissue type and other information are registered with UK Transplant. This is a NHS organization in Bristol which keeps a list of all patients awaiting kidney transplantation. Similar organizations exist in other parts of the world.

When a suitable kidney donor dies, the tissue type and blood group are notified to UK Transplant, where a computer finds the two most suitable recipients amongst those on the waiting list.

Sources of Kidneys for Transplantation

Only human kidneys are suitable for transplantation into humans. It has been found that kidneys transplanted from animals to man are rapidly rejected.

Two types of human kidneys are used in transplantation – cadaver kidneys and live donor kidneys. A cadaver kidney is obtained from a previously fit person who has just died as a result of a road accident or some sudden illness. The majority of kidneys transplanted in Great Britain are cadaver kidneys. A live donor kidney is removed from a healthy relative or friend of the person with chronic renal failure. A kidney may be transplanted from a parent or from a brother or sister. Sometimes cousins prove to be suitable donors. There is always a shortage of kidneys for transplantation. When it was appreciated how powerfully cyclosporin can control rejection of kidneys a number of American surgeons reasoned that it would be justifiable to transplant kidneys from non-related donors provided that the donor was an adult, mature and well motivated. A new expression was coined – the 'living non-related donor'. Thus, provided that the blood group was identical a husband could donate a kidney to his wife and vice versa. Further, in principle, friends of dialysis patients could donate kidneys. This is a new topic and adequate long term experience is not yet available to evaluate it fully.

When a potential donor decides to offer a kidney for transplantation he or she is carefully checked. This includes physical examination, tests of blood and urine, X-rays of the kidneys and also testing as far as possible that the donor kidney will not be rejected by the recipient. If all tests are satisfactory the transplant operation can be planned. The ideal live donor kidney is obtained from the identical twin of the recipient. This type of kidney is the most likely to work well for a number of years.

Preparation for the Operation

Cadaver kidneys will only remain suitable for transplantation up to 30 hours after removal from the donor. There may be little or no warning that a potential donor is about to die. The blood group and tissue type of the donor are reported to the UK Transplant in Bristol where they are compared with the tissue types of patients awaiting transplant and the two most suitable recipients are selected. One donor has two kidneys, which can be transplanted into two separate people who may be in different parts of the country. The recipient's doctors are then notified and in turn the patient himself is informed and comes to hospital. Because donor and recipient may be at opposite ends of the country the kidney may have to be transported many miles in a short time. When the donor kidney is received at the transplant unit, testing of donor blood cells against the potential recipient's blood has to be completed. This takes a few hours. By the time donor-recipient compatibility is confirmed there may be little time left before the transplant must be performed. Thus the recipient may have a very short notice of his operation. In some cases there may be warning that a potential donor is about to die. The necessary tissue typing and blood grouping may then be done within usual working hours. The recipient will have a little more warning of the operation and need not rush to hospital.

The period of waiting for a matching kidney to become available may be months or years during which the patient is maintained on dialysis. For the patient who is to receive a kidney from a live donor the operation is planned a few weeks ahead. Tissue typing and matching are carried out before the operation is decided upon. The patient is dialysed the day before transplantation.

The sequence of events before a cadaver kidney transplant varies slightly in different hospitals. The following is a broad outline of what a patient should do.

(1) Make sure that the renal unit has your correct address and phone numbers so that you can be contacted at work or at home, day and night.

(2) At holidays or if away for a few days inform the transplant ward staff of the temporary telephone number and address. It is a shame to miss the chance of a transplant because of a short break.

(3) Keep an overnight bag packed. Pyjamas or nightdress, dressing gown, toiletries and something to read are required.

(4) Make arrangements for the care of children or pets in your sudden absence. A patient will be in hospital about 2 to 3 weeks; sometimes longer.

(5) Warn your employer or employees of a possible sudden operation.

When telephoned that a kidney is available that may 'fit' you, the points following are useful:

(1) Hurry; time is often short at this stage.

(2) Do not eat or drink. It is dangerous to have a general anaesthetic with food or fluid in the stomach.

(3) If you drive to hospital have someone to accompany you to take the car away after your arrival. Not all hospitals have parking spaces for patients and none will accept the responsibility for such vehicles.

(4) If, by chance you happen to have a cold or are unwell for any other reason, tell the nurse who telephones you. This will save time and disappointment; a person is not transplanted if he has even a mild infection.

Pre-transplant Blood Transfusion

There is no doubt that kidney graft survival is improved if the patient has received two or more blood transfusions well before the operation. The reason for this improvement is not known but the effect is important. Some people are concerned that a blood transfusion may transmit an infection – in particular the AIDS virus. All blood before transfusion is now tested for this virus and other possible infections. Blood transfusion is now very safe and should not cause anxiety.

The Transplant Operation

If the tests of donor blood cells against the patient's blood show that the potential kidney will 'fit' then the operation is 'on'.

Once it has been decided to perform the transplant the following events occur:

(1) The patient undresses, is examined by a doctor and gives consent for the operation.

(2) Blood is taken for a few pre-operative tests.

(3) A chest x-ray is taken and an ECG is performed.

(4) If necessary a short haemodialysis will be performed. For people on CAPD, fluid is run out of the abdomen and no fresh sample is run in.

(5) The patient is shaved from nipple to knee, has a bath or shower and puts on a hospital gown. Dentures are removed, valuables and cash are kept safely by nursing staff.

(6) About one hour before the operation an injection is given which makes the person drowsy and relaxed. He then rests in bed until taken to the operating theatre.

The graft kidney is placed in the lower right or left portion of the abdomen as shown in Figure 16.1. This position for the graft kidney is chosen because the operation is simpler. The surgeon sews the artery of the new kidney to an artery in the pelvis. The donor renal vein is sewn to a vein in the pelvis. In this way blood flows to and from the kidney and it may commence to make urine straight away. The next step in the operation is to connect the donor ureter (the tube through which urine passes) to the bladder. The wound is then sewn up. The operation takes about four hours. A catheter is placed in the bladder so that the volume

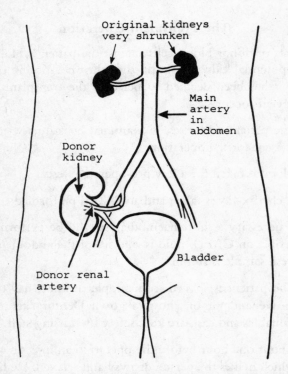

Figure 16.1 The position in which a transplant kidney is placed. The patient is often able to feel the new kidney in the lower right or left part of the abdomen

of urine produced can be accurately measured. It is removed after four to seven days.

The patient is returned to the ward and remembers little of the next 12 or so hours because of the effects of the anaesthetic. He is usually nursed in a cubicle. One or two 'drips' (intravenous infusions) will have been set up whilst in theatre and are removed one or two days after the operation. At this stage eating is possible and necessary to speed recovery. For the first few days pulse, temperature, blood pressure and urine are all checked frequently. The drugs used to prevent kidney rejection are given at regular times. The abdomen is sore for the first two days but the patient will be eased out of bed on the first post-operative day and by the third day will be walking. Visitors are allowed after the first 24 hours. Quite frequently after a successful transplant the patient's fistula clots spontaneously. This is a normal event related to the improved haemoglobin which is a consequence of a healthy kidney (page 26).

Many transplanted kidneys produce urine at the time of operation or begin to function 24–48 hours afterwards. Some kidneys are damaged temporarily during storage before grafting and may take a week or more before urine production begins. It may therefore be necessary to haemodialyse a person a few times after the transplant operation before kidney function begins. For the CAPD patient, CAPD is performed by nursing staff until the transplant works. The period of waiting until a transplant kidney begins to function may be an anxious time for the patient and his relatives. There are tests to show if the kidney is healing or not. A slow start does not reduce the potential long-term function of the kidney.

It takes a few days to recover from the operation. After this the patient is taught to measure and to make a note of his urine output over each 24 hours. This, like taking the drugs regularly, is essential so that if the flow of urine diminishes the cause can be rapidly diagnosed. Most transplant units take this opportunity to teach the patient about drugs and how often they need to be taken. It is essential that the patient understands these matters because if the drugs are forgotten it is quite probable that the kidney will be rejected.

Reduction in flow of urine is important because in the first few weeks after a transplant, perhaps while the patient is still in hospital, it may well be caused by acute rejection of the grafted kidney. Other symptoms which may occur in this condition are a feeling of being unwell, fever, a rise in the pulse rate and perhaps tenderness of the kidney. The treatment is straightforward and comprises injections of prednisolone into a vein. Usually the acute rejection is reversed within a day or so. The volume of urine increases and the other symptoms go. Acute rejection is a common occurrence. Most patients suffer only one episode, but some patients experience more. An acute rejection, correctly treated, does not affect the long term survival of the kidney.

Follow Up after Transplantation

A patient leaves hospital about three weeks after the operation. He is seen regularly and at first frequently in an out-patient clinic. For the first few weeks a recipient usually attends three times a week. At this early stage the risk of acute rejection is still present. If the patient is checked frequently it is possible to diagnose the rejection early which leads to prompt successful treatment.

If there is doubt about kidney function after discharge from hospital it may be necessary for the patient to attend daily or perhaps to be readmitted for a few days. Many episodes of acute rejection are treated without re-admission.

With the passage of time and increasing stability of function, visits to transplant out-patients can be less frequent. At each visit blood pressure and graft kidney function are measured. Changes in drug dose are made if required. Assuming good health visits are only required at monthly intervals and later every three months. The amount of time involved with a transplant is quite considerable: at least three months off work are necessary.

Results of Transplantation

A transplanted kidney does not work for ever. How long a donor kidney works depends in part upon the type of kidney. The survival times of three different types of donor kidneys are shown in Figure 16.2. The information needed to draw this graph was obtained from many transplant units in Europe and before the beneficial effects of cyclosporin became widely available. The precise percentage survival of the kidneys transplanted is not the same in each unit. There are many technical reasons for this.

Figure 16.2 shows that the ideal donor kidney comes from an identical twin. The survival of these kidneys is better than that of a kidney from a non-twin relative or cadaver donor. Identical twins are not very common and therefore transplantation of a kidney from an identical twin to another is infrequent.

If a suitable kidney can be obtained from a close relative of the patient it is likely to work longer than a cadaver kidney. However

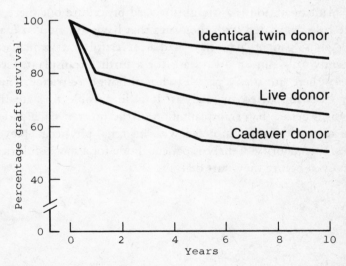

Figure 16.2   A graph showing the average survival of three different types of transplant kidneys

133

in Britain most families are small and it is usually difficult to find a suitable donor from a brother, sister or parent. The majority of kidneys grafted in Britain are from cadavers. Figure 16.2 shows about 30% of all these kidneys have failed by one year after the operation. These unfortunate people return to dialysis and, if they wish it, are put on the UK Transplant list for a further graft kidney. For those people with functioning cadaver kidneys one year after operation the outlook is fairly good. Their graft kidneys may well work for a number of years during which they can enjoy a near normal life. Many live donor and cadaver kidneys function for more than ten years.

Home Dialysis versus Transplantation

This may be a difficult choice to make. Home dialysis (haemo-dialysis, CAPD or CCPD) is a very safe, effective, longterm treatment of chronic renal failure but there are regular chores associated with these types of dialysis (pages 85 and 114). A transplant operation is a straightforward procedure but there are some risks associated with the drugs that have to be taken (page 122). Those patients who have had a successful graft which subsequently fails almost always ask for a further transplant. Conversely there are many people who, although restricted, enjoy their lives supported by dialysis. It is impossible to state that dialysis is better than transplantation or the reverse. Each patient must discuss the topic in detail with his renal physician. Nevertheless the majority of dialysis patients hope for a successful transplant even before they start dialysis.

17

The transplant co-ordinator

As mentioned in the previous chapter, the majority of kidneys transplanted are obtained from a person who has recently died. Since it is neither practicable nor legal for one doctor to be responsible for the care of a dying patient together with undertaking the organisation of removal and transplantation of the kidneys, co-ordinators have been appointed to help this delicate, urgent and important work.

Transplant Co-ordinators

Kidneys are transplanted in only 31 hospitals in Great Britain. Organs for transplantation become available from a much greater number of hospitals. It follows that there is a need for specially trained people to work between hospitals where donor kidneys become available and transplant units. This is the task of the transplant co-ordinator. Many co-ordinators have been transplant ward sisters because the co-ordinator must have detailed knowledge of all aspects of the subject. A co-ordinator may be attached to one or more transplant units: a system is devised to share kidneys between the transplant hospitals concerned or, if a suitable patient is not available, to offer the kidney to U.K. Transplant (page 125). The co-ordinators are also involved with the transplantation of hearts, lungs and livers in addition to kidneys. These different types of transplant are performed in different hospitals: hence it may be difficult and time consuming to arrange the prompt removal of the various organs by the separate transplant teams. Because people do not die at any particular time a co-ordinator works very long irregular hours and must be available continuously for long periods of time.

The Transplant Co-ordinator's Job

This important work requires much commonsense, tact and ability to get on well with hospital staff of differing seniorities, patients and relatives.

The central feature of a co-ordinator's job is to obtain kidneys and other organs for transplantation. In this way the person who has suddenly died is able to contribute to the health of others which in itself is a comfort to the bereaved. In some wards nursing and medical staff change fairly frequently and regularly. Some of them may be unaware of the shortage of transplant kidneys. Co-ordinators make regular visits talking about different aspects of transplantation. Other staff while being aware that transplantation is important may not know of the most suitable type of donor, how to approach relatives or how to contact transplant staff. Here the expert co-ordinator supplies the necessary information about a potential donor and is able to speak to his or her relatives if required. With knowledge of transplantation, its advantages, how and when organs are removed she is able to set relatives minds at rest.

One further important task is the education of the general public concerning the persistent need for transplant organs. Thus a co-ordinator may speak at meetings of interested groups and encourage the carrying of organ donor cards.

The Value of Transplant Co-ordinators

Table 17.1 shows the numbers of patients waiting for a transplant and the number performed in Great Britain from 1979 to 1986. There is no doubt that the gradual increase in transplants is due to the efforts of the co-ordinators. As yet there are insufficient employed. Worryingly, the number of people who hope for a transplant is increasing more rapidly than the number of kidneys transplanted. This means that more patients are waiting longer on haemodialysis or one of the types of peritoneal dialysis. This is disappointing for the people concerned, causes congestion in renal units and is increasingly expensive for the National Health Service. The gap between those hoping for a graft and those gaining a new kidney can only be closed by the hard work of transplant co-ordinators.

Table 17.1   The number of patients awaiting a transplant and the number performed from 1979 to 1986 in Great Britain. Figures have been rounded to the nearest 10. (Information by courtesy of Dr B.A. Bradley, Director UK Transplant Service)

Year	Patients waiting	Transplants performed
1979	1590	840
1980	1920	930
1981	2270	850
1982	2480	1090
1983	2610	1180
1984	2780	1550
1985	3440	1430
1986	3470	1580

Conclusion

In the last 15 years there have been four important forward steps in kidney transplantation. They are: pre-transplant blood transfusion (page 129), the use of cyclosporin (page 123), possibly better tissue matching (page 120) and the appointment of transplant co–ordinators.

18

Survival on dialysis and transplantation

This topic may frequently cross the minds of patients, their relatives and friends. At the beginning of the chapter it must be emphasized that only broad outlines and generalities can be discussed. Direct application to an individual is not possible. A patient needing specific information because of family responsibilities or other reasons should ask his renal physician. However, even then an informed guess is all that can be offered.

It is obvious that a patient starting dialysis aged 20 years will almost certainly live longer than a similar person commencing aged 75 years. Likewise a person with a disease affecting only the kidneys will probably survive longer than a patient of the same age but with a generalised disease which involves other organs as well as the kidneys. People who look after themselves carefully probably will enjoy more years than those who sometimes require emergency dialysis for fluid overload (page 101) or hyperkalaemia (pages 19 and 100). People develop terminal renal failure at any age. Raised blood pressure is common in people with progressive renal failure. If found early and correctly treated the strain upon the heart and blood vessels is reduced. Increased blood pressure itself causes no symptoms and may only be detected at a later stage. There are two forms of dialysis; both haemodialysis and peritoneal dialysis have separate problems related to the form of treatment. When a patient receives a transplant kidney, dialysis difficulties are behind him, but these are exchanged for a slight but distinct risk of infection which may be fatal. The length of survival of a person treated in a renal unit varies according to the age at beginning of dialysis, to a slight extent to the type of dialysis used, the disease which caused terminal renal failure, whether a transplant is performed and how well the person is able to adapt to differing circumstances.

Figure 18.1 outlines the major events which may occur to someone who has progressive renal failure which reaches terminal renal failure. Terminal renal failure is fatal if the person is not dialysed. Features favouring survival on dialysis and after transplantation will be discussed.

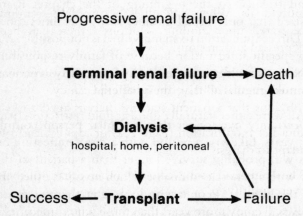

Figure 18.1   The sequence of events which may occur to a patient who develops terminal renal failure

Long-term Dialysis Survival

Most information is available concerning haemodialysis because long-term peritoneal dialysis is a relatively new development. Nevertheless, it appears that haemodialysis and CAPD are equally successful for at least 5 years – it is too soon to know if the benefits of CAPD extend longer but there is no obvious reason why this should not be so. In 1986 two American patients were presented with awards for having continued with CAPD for 8 years. There are a few patients who have been treated with haemodialysis for more than 20 years. By the mid 1980s it became not uncommon for patients to pass their 15th year of haemodialysis. Features which they had in common were:

(1) They began therapy whilst being 20–40 years old.

(2) They either had mild hypertension or if severely raised blood pressure it had been well and persistently treated.

(3) All were mature cheerful, outgoing, adaptable, resourceful individuals. When difficulties occurred their minds concentrated upon finding solutions rather than becoming depressed and anxious.

(4) None were cigarette smokers. Haemodialysis patients who smoke regularly halve their life expectancy.

(5) All were either naturally good at fluid restriction (page 100) and diet modification (page 104) or rapidly learnt how to adapt to dialysis.

(6) They only had kidney disease, other organs of their body were healthy.

Therefore, in general terms, those who will probably die sooner have one or more of the following features or conditions:

(1) Old age.

(2) Severe uncontrolled or poorly controlled blood pressure.

The heart is persistently strained, there is a risk of a heart attack or stroke.

(3) Those who are unable or who do not wish to face their future in a determined, positive way.

(4) Those who smoke cigarettes.

(5) Those who take too much fluid between haemodialysis may risk their lives. A weight gain of 3–5 kg (6–12 lb) above the 'dry weight' (page 101) is dangerous, can be very unpleasant and possibly fatal. Some people have killed themselves by eating too many foods which are high in potassium (page 100).

(6) It is particularly unfortunate if a person develops terminal renal failure and the underlying disease continues to destroy other organs. The commonest example is diabetes mellitus. After dialysis has begun, damage to blood vessels elsewhere in the body continues. Diabetics must take particular care of themselves. Happily CAPD leads to a very good control of blood sugar (page 85).

Features Favouring a Healthy Life on Peritoneal Dialysis

As stated on page 141 less long-term information is available concerning CAPD, CCPD and IPD. Nevertheless general points are clear and apply to each type of peritoneal dialysis:

(1) The patient who mentally and physically adapts in a purposeful manner will enjoy a better and perhaps longer life than a person who is poorly motivated.

(2) Apart from the discomfort and inconvenience of recurrent episodes of peritonitis (page 85) the peritoneum may be damaged and can lead to failure of this form of dialysis.

(3) As for haemodialysis patients fluid restriction is required. While it is possible to 'suck out' extra fluid with 'strong

bags' (page 55) their excessive use is not a good habit.

(4) Persistent cigarette smoking leads to an earlier death.

Prolonged Survival after a Kidney Transplant

There are a few patients who have functioning grafts which were transplanted more than 20 years ago. The numbers are small because not many transplants were performed at that time and few grafts function for such long periods.

Transplants fail for many reasons; the majority of which are no fault of the recipient. However the patient can help himself towards better health.

(1) Drugs to prevent rejection must be taken every day and in some cases at a particular time of the day. The transplant recipient who goes away for a weekend leaving the necessary drugs at home will develop an acute rejection and it may be impossible to save the kidney.

(2) Appetite is increased when taking prednisolone (page 122). There is a possibility of becoming too fat. Obesity is unhealthy. The dietician can help with avoiding this hazard (page 103).

(3) The drugs used to prevent kidney rejection render the person slightly more prone to infection. Thus if a person thinks that infection is developing he should telephone his transplant unit without delay. Remaining at home 'hoping it will get better' is unwise.

Why Transplant Kidneys Fail

Approximate survival of different types of transplanted kidneys is shown in Figure 16.2, page 133. Clearly the majority of people can confidently expect a useful number of dialysis-free years after a successful transplant kidney. There are two types of transplant kidney failure: either only the kidney and the patient then returns to dialysis or complete failure when the patient dies.

Kidney Failure

Chronic rejection is the commonest cause of graft kidney failure. It is not known why this occurs and no specific treatment is available. Over a period of years the graft gradually scars and the person develops chronic renal failure again (page 133). Perhaps the use of cyclosporin may diminish the frequency of chronic rejection but it is too soon to be certain.

Stopping anti–rejection drugs guarantees loss of the transplant kidney (page 143).

Much less common causes of transplant failure are recurrence of the person's original nephritis in the transplant kidney. If the person is diabetic, then diabetic kidney failure may develop.

The renal artery or vein of the transplant may become blocked with blood clot. There is no treatment: the graft is then removed.

Patient Death

Death of a transplant recipient because of the graft is infrequent. The causes in approximate order of frequency are:

(1) Infection. Frequently this is sudden and can be impossible to cure. Any part of the body may be affected. Infections involving the blood, lung, heart together with abscesses are well known.

(2) Heart attacks or strokes may occur but probably related to previous high blood pressure. The risk is the same for patients receiving haemodialysis or peritoneal dialysis.

(3) Years of treatment with prednisolone and azathioprine very slightly increase the chance of the patient developing a specific type of malignancy. The probability for a patient is minimal because even in a busy transplant centre such an event may only occur once every 10 years. Whether this risk

is true for people taking cyclosporin is, as yet, unknown.

(4) The transplant operation itself is very safe. Death directly caused by the surgery or anaesthetic is almost unknown.

Because of the above reasons, there are anxieties associated with kidney transplantation. Nevertheless, a large majority of kidney patients think of a 'new' kidney as the best treatment of terminal renal failure.

Conclusion

For the first ten years or so there is little difference in survival for patients receiving a transplant or choosing long-term home haemodialysis. Chronic peritoneal dialysis may prove equally successful. At present longest survival is gained from haemodialysis. Whether cyclosporin will improve very long-term transplant survival is unknown.

19

Social service support

Unfortunately not everyone treated with regular dialysis is able to work full-time. Some people are unable to find any employment. Fortunately the State provides a number of benefits which are available to dialysis and transplant patients. This short chapter is a general guide for patients in Great Britain. Help is available from two main sources. Firstly staff of the local branch of the Department of Health and Social Security should be able to supply advice regarding benefits and how to claim them. Secondly all local authorities have Citizens' Advice Bureaux where staff are expert in advising and helping people and they keep up-to-date in changes in regulations. A visit is recommended. Every renal unit has a social worker who is able to advise in general terms regarding benefits and has a much wider role which includes discussion of, and help with, difficult or delicate matters. As well as social workers based in the hospital, each local authority has a Social Service department to provide advice and support to people in the local community.

The sums of money that a person may claim are not stated

because the rates of benefit vary from time to time with changes in legislation.

Benefits Available

There are comprehensive benefits available which may be helpful if a person loses income because of illness. The main benefits are as follows:

Attendance Allowance

If help is needed long-term to wash, dress, feed or to ensure a person's safety the attendance allowance may be payable. Details are given in the DHSS leaflet NI 205 'Attendance Allowance'.

Mobility Allowance

This is payable to people less than 75 years of age if they have difficulty in walking a modest distance. The allowance is paid regardless of income and permits the person concerned to car tax exemption and some parking concessions. The DHSS leaflet NI 2111 'Mobility Allowance' gives the details.

Statutory Sick Pay

This sum is paid by an employer for the first 8 weeks of sickness in any tax year provided that the employee has previously paid Class 1 National Insurance contributions. The sum is proportional to the individual's average weekly earnings. The DHSS leaflet NI 244 should be consulted.

Sickness Benefit

This benefit is more complex and is best explained by the personnel of a Citizens' Advice Bureau. In principle money is available for as long as 28 weeks or for 20 weeks after Statutory Sick Pay expires. An introduction to this complex topic is given in the DHSS leaflet NI 16 'Statutory Sick Pay & Sickness Benefit'.

Invalidity Benefit

Again this is relatively complex and expert advice is useful. Invalidity Benefit exists for those people who still require help after the 28th week of Sickness Benefit has been paid. This benefit provides long-term financial aid for the chronically ill. The DHSS leaflet NI 16A and the local Citizens' Advice Bureau should be consulted.

Supplementary Benefit

If the above benefits, perhaps together with part-time earnings are insufficient to live on, a patient may claim Supplementary Benefit (Leaflet SB1). To claim Supplementary Benefit a patient's savings must be less than £3000. Any special needs of the claimant are taken into account. These may include:

(1) Extra heating that may be required.

(2) Additional expense because of a diet prescribed on medical grounds.

(3) Laundry expenses.

The Family Income Supplement is claimable by people who work full-time for low wages and are bringing up children. The same additional benefits are available to those who qualify for the Family Income Supplement as for those people who get the Supplementary Benefit.

Prescription Charges

Kidney patients usually need regular drugs and the prescription charges may easily add up to several pounds each month.

Before dialysis a patient does not qualify for free drugs unless a chronic non-kidney disease is also present. Such diseases include diabetes or thyroid gland failure. The majority of people have to pay the prescription charges for the medicines they need. The prepayment or 'season ticket' system is good value for money for the patient receiving three or more drugs prescribed monthly. The necessary form is available from the local NHS Family Practitioner Committee Office or the Health Board Office in Scotland.

Dialysis patients have automatic exemption from all prescription charges.

Transplant patients. The DHSS does not automatically exempt these patients from prescription charges.

People in receipt of Supplementary Benefit automatically qualify for free NHS prescriptions, spectacles and dental treatment. It is well worth consulting pamphlets P11, G11 and D11 respectively.

Miscellaneous Allowances

The following are general guides and a person who may qualify should obtain the appropriate leaflet and discuss the matter with someone in the local Citizens' Advice Bureau or his social worker.

Tax rebates

People who are unemployed for more than four weeks and have been paying PAYE can claim tax rebates. Form P50 has to be filled in and returned to the Inland Revenue.

Rent and rate allowance or rebate
A dialysis patient is eligible to apply for the above if he is not receiving Supplementary Benefit. Details are available from the Housing Department of the local Council Offices.

Attendance allowance
This benefit is payable to home haemodialysis patients to allow them to pay someone to help them when on dialysis. It is tax-free and is claimable by using Leaflet NI205.

Parking permits for disabled
These permits allow a patient to park his car without charge or time limit at a parking meter and to park on single yellow lines for up to two hours. Renal patients do not automatically qualify for one of these permits. Advice is available from Social Services Departments and from Council Offices.

Travelling expenses
Travelling is expensive; help may be available

(1) For patients receiving Supplementary Benefit travel costs are refunded at the hospital upon production of the current Allowance Book.

(2) For people not receiving either of the above supplements money may be available to pay fares to and from hospital if the patient has a low income. Form H11 is available from hospitals and after completion has to be sent to the local Social Security Office.

Rate reduction
For people who own their own homes in which a room has been converted for dialysis a reduction in the rateable value may be possible. The Rates Office has to be contacted: the address can be obtained from the Town Hall.

Telephone and electricity
For patients on home dialysis the hospital will pay for electricity used in the dialysis room and telephone rental charges.

Conclusion

There are a number of different ways in which the State can help the kidney patient. There are many leaflets covering the benefits which may be claimed. These make rather daunting reading. It is a complicated subject and a patient should start by talking to the medical social worker of the renal unit concerned or to a member of the staff of the local Citizens' Advice Bureau who will be able to guide him through the maze.

20

History of dialysis and transplantation

Because you will be dependent upon an artificial kidney or peritoneal dialysis for some time, it may be of interest to read something about the development of these kinds of treatments. This is a short account of the way in which the practices of dialysis and transplantation have developed and grown over the years.

Haemodialysis

Renal medicine is a relatively new subject. In the early 1940s Dr W.J. Kolff, working in Nazi-dominated Holland, developed the first artificial kidney. By present-day standards it was very cumbersome and tedious to use. Kolff's idea and the work stemming from it were the major steps forward in the treatment of kidney disease during the first fifty years of this century. The principle by which his machine worked is still in use in all present-day haemodialysis machines.

After the Second World War Kolff gave a number of his artificial kidneys to major hospitals in Europe and America. The first artificial kidney arrived in Great Britain in 1946. It was used, as were all the machines of that period, for the treatment of people who developed acute renal failure during the course of severe illnesses where return of normal renal function could be expected after the illness. The treatment of chronic renal failure by dialysis as it is understood today was not then thought of.

During the late 1940s and the early 1950s technical advances in the design of artificial kidneys were made but very few people received treatment. The Korean war (1950–53) provided a stimulus to the use of the artificial kidney. Modified Kolff kidneys were used in field hospitals where kidney failure occurred as a complication of war wounds. At that time there was not a great deal of interest in chronic dialysis and only a few groups of private individuals continued making improvements in the design of artificial kidneys. At this time all artificial kidneys consisted of a large drum which was covered by a semipermeable membrane of cellulose acetate, thus providing a large surface area over which blood from the patient was brought into contact with dialysate. Across the semipermeable membrane waste products would pass from the patient's blood into the dialysate. Dr A. MacNeil in America had the idea of using several layers of cellulose acetate like a sandwich, the 'filling' of which was alternately blood and dialysate. In this way a large surface area of membrane was arranged more compactly. Many present-day dialysers are designed on modifications of this clever idea, which made the artificial kidney much less cumbersome. Nowadays the term artificial kidney is used loosely to cover the complete apparatus used for haemodialysis. Strictly the artificial kidney is only that part containing the semipermeable membrane and is more correctly called the dialyser. The other parts of the haemodialysis machine include pumps and monitoring systems.

Interest in dialysis for the treatment of acute renal failure gradually increased in the 1950s. The first unit in Great Britain was in Leeds, led by Dr F. M. Parsons.

The major difficulty of those days was the lack of a satisfactory system for taking blood from and then returning it to the patient. This problem prevented the development of chronic dialysis because it is not possible to dialyse a person repeatedly using his normal unmodified arteries and veins. The blood vessels clot when used a number of times and then cannot be used again. In 1960 an important contribution to dialysis was made by Dr B. Scribner of the University of Washington. He and his colleague Quinton developed the first adequate shunt. A shunt is an artificial connection between an artery and a vein in two halves which can be separated for dialysis (see page 48). The tube attached to the artery is used to lead blood to the machine. Blood is returned from the machine to the patient through the tube connected to the vein. When not being used for dialysis the two ends of the shunt are joined together. Silicone rubber is used for the connection because it is sufficiently flexible to allow the patient to move his arm without causing damage to the vessels into which the shunt is secured. Scribner then set up the first chronic dialysis unit in the United States.

In London, in 1961, Dr S. Shaldon taught the first patient in the world to dialyse himself. By 1964 Shaldon's group had established the first person on home dialysis. During the remainder of the 1960s chronic dialysis expanded rapidly in Britain, Europe and America. The handful of units in Britain grew and there are now more than sixty.

The main problems of the Scribner shunt are clotting or infection, or both. Some of these shunts worked for years, but most survived only for months. The patients then had to enter hospital for a new shunt to be inserted.

In 1966 a new approach to gain access to the blood circulation was described by Dr J. Cimino of New York. His idea was simple and the results were good. A vein in the forearm was sewn to the artery that runs down towards the base of the thumb. Some of the blood that previously flowed to the hand passed directly into that vein. In time the vein grew larger due to the increased quantity of blood passing through it. A direct connection between an artery and a vein using no artificial tube is called a fistula. It was then possible to put wide-bore needles into the Cimino fistula to carry blood to and from the dialyser every time dialysis was required (see page 50). The use of fistulae has totally replaced shunts for chronic haemodialysis patients.

During the 1970s there was a steady improvement in the design of dialysis machines and dialysers. Disposable dialysers became widely used. In the 1980s there has been a trend away from parallel flow dialysers towards the hollow fibre type. Many are washed and sterilised after dialysis and then re-used six or more times.

Disposable dialysers are more efficient than the older type so it has been possible to shorten the number of hours of dialysis per week. In 1970 an average patient was dialysed about 30 hours per week. It is now about 10–14 hours, divided into two or three periods.

Peritoneal Dialysis

The alternative to haemodialysis for the treatment of chronic renal failure is peritoneal dialysis. A tube, called a catheter, is put into the belly through a small cut just by the navel. The lining of the body cavity and covering the intestines is called the peritoneum, and works as a semipermeable membrane. Dialysate is run into the abdomen through the catheter. Over a period of time waste products cross the peritoneum from the bloodstream into the dialysate which is then allowed to flow back out of the body through the catheter (see page 55).

This technique began in the early 1960s but because the catheters then in use were rigid and uncomfortable they could not be used repeatedly. A big improvement was made by Dr H. Tenckhoff in 1968. He developed a flexible non-irritating catheter which is inserted into the abdomen and can be used again and again for years. This advance encouraged the development of semi-automatic peritoneal dialysis machines which can be used at home or in hospital. The dialysis is slow but gentle and a number of people are being treated in this way.

The most recent development in peritoneal dialysis is the so-called continuous ambulatory peritoneal dialysis (CAPD). It was devised by Dr R. Popovich in 1976 and uses the Tenckhoff catheter. The procedure is easy to learn, allows mobility during dialysis and gives a good quality life. CAPD became feasible in 1980 when dialysate was first supplied in plastic bags which could be folded and tucked into the clothing. The number of patients on CAPD grew most rapidly in Great Britain in the first few years of the 1980s. The system is now very popular world-wide and used for about half of all dialysis patients. In Great Britain and other countries CAPD has allowed doctors to treat people in their sixties and seventies who otherwise would never have gained the chance of dialysis.

Transplantation

The first successful human kidney transplant operation was performed in Chicago in 1950. The kidney worked for nine months. The first transplant from one identical twin to the other was in 1954. This operation was very successful and showed the long-term value of kidney grafts. Problems occurred when kidneys were transplanted into people who were not the identical twin of the person who gave the kidney. Very frequently the transplanted kidney was rejected shortly after the operation and its ability to produce urine and to purify the blood was lost. In 1959 in Boston and in Paris it was found that if patients were treated with X-rays before transplant operation the kidney was much less likely to be rejected. It was not easy to judge the correct dose of X-rays – if too large there was a danger of serious infection and if too small the kidney might well be rejected.

In 1961 Professor R. Y. Calne of Cambridge found that the drug azathioprine (Imuran) was very powerful in slowing down kidney rejection in dogs. The same beneficial results were found in humans. This discovery led to a gradual increase in the number and success of kidney transplantation operations. During the second half of the 1960s the number of dialysis units and therefore of patients on dialysis in Britain increased considerably. There was therefore a much increased need for donor kidneys. The supply of kidneys is always less than the demand. Transplant surgeons and renal physicians make repeated efforts to obtain adequate numbers of kidneys but are relatively unsuccessful. Many patients have to wait years for a suitable kidney. The supply of donor kidneys has not improved in recent years and is still inadequate. This may improve if the unrelated donor scheme (page 126) catches on widely.

In the late 1960s the techniques of tissue typing were developed so that more precise matching of donor kidneys to the proposed recipient became possible. In 1972 the National Health Service set up the UK Transplant service in Bristol. Details of each potential kidney transplant patient in the country are kept on computer file. When a donor kidney becomes available the blood group tissue type are then telephoned to UK Transplant. The computer identifies the patient who would be the most suitable recipient. Arrangements are made to transport the kidney from the hospital where it was obtained to the transplant centre where it will be used. Many countries have set up similar organisations to aid kidney transplantation.

In the 1970s it was found that blood transfusions to the recipient months before the transplant operation improve the length of survival of the donor kidney.

The most exciting development in transplantation was the introduction of cyclosporin – a powerful anti-rejection drug. While complicated to use, survival of transplant kidneys has increased by at least 10 per cent at all stages. Professor Calne was one of the principal innovators of the use of this drug.

The Future of Dialysis and Transplantation

From the above short history it is obvious that renal medicine has made very rapid progress. Probably more efficient artificial kidneys will be developed and perhaps the hours of dialysis will be shortened further. CAPD will continue to be used widely for people of all ages and for diabetics. The greatest need at present is to increase the number of kidneys obtained for transplant so that the most suitable match can be made for patients. The long-term aim is for the grafted kidney to function in its new owner for as long as the person lives.

Index

INDEX

renal unit, composition of 65–6
Resonium 62
Rocaltrol 61
run-in time 20

saline 20, 66
salt, dietary 105
scarred kidney 33, 36
Scribner, B., *see* Quinton–Scribner
    shunt
semi-permeable membrane 20, 43–6
    salt movement 44–6
    waste diffusion 43–4
sexual activity 39–40, 75–6, 86, 107–
    8, 121
shunt 20, 48–9, 58, 72, 155
    clotting 72, 155
    Quinton–Scribner 20, 48–9, 155
Sickness Benefit 149
smoking, *see* cigarettes
social services 147–52
Statutory Sick Pay 148
sterile 20, 66, 68, 92
stones, kidney 34–5
Supplementary Benefit 149–50
survival 133–4, 142

tax rebates 150
technical terms, *see* dialysis; glossary
    of technical terms
telephone, for home dialysis 110–
    112, 143, 152
Tenckhoff catheter, *see* catheter
tissue types 21, 120–1, 127, 138
transplant co-ordinator 135–8
    job of 136
    value of 137
transplantation 119–34
    advantages of 121
    blood transfusion before 129, 138
    disadvantages 121–2
    drugs and 122–4
    failure of 143–5
    in females 108
    follow-up 132
    history of 157–9
    home dialysis and 134

kidney sources 126
    operation 129–32
    preparation for 127–8
    success of 133–4
    UK Transplant service 158
    waiting list for 125, 137
travel, and dialysis, *see* holidays
travelling expenses 151
twins 126, 133

ultrafiltration 21, 44, 50, 70
under-dialysis 21, 72–3
United Kingdom Transplant
    service 158
urea 21, 59–60
ureter 21, 24, 35–6
    stones in 35
urethra 24–5, 35–6
    male 37
urinary tract 21, 23
    anatomy 23–5
urine 25–7
    amounts 25, 27, 29, 41, 59,
        132
    flow obstruction 34, 37
    measuring 131
    nocturnal 38–9, 41
    reflux 35–6
    transplantation and flow 131
USA 12

vascular access 21
vitamins 61, 98–9
vomiting 39, 73

'wash back' 22, 70
'washed-out' 22, 73–4
water
    foods and 27
    soft 20
    see also fluids
weight
    'dry' 70
    loss 92
    'wet' 68
    see also obesity